Printed in the United States of America

ISBN-13:
978-1539303084

ISBN-10:
153930308X

Acknowledgements

Thank you...

...Mom, for the encouragement to dream.

...Dad, for the work ethic that does not quit.

...Siseff, for the laughter and support that can only be provided by the greatest sister and best friend I could ever hope for.

...Nick and "Mayo", for sharing your fitness knowledge and the constant coaching through some of the toughest times in my life.

...Vee, Janet, Dustin, & Kate, for putting up with my version of humor, sharing life experiences with me, and teaching me to enjoy the journey.

...Mike, Chris, John, & Kate H., for taking the time to share your knowledge so openly, believing that it would be a good investment of your time, and guiding me through such valuable lessons in life.

...Rachel, Steven, and Sammy J., for inspiring me to become a better trainer.

...clients, for your trust, laughing with me, and believing in my lessons...ok, and the sass.

Introduction

As a newly certified Personal Trainer back in 2012, it was my responsibility at the fitness club to introduce new members to our club and at times, introduce the new members to the basics of wellness by providing New Member Assessments. During these hour(ish)-long sessions, I was expected to cover *some* information regarding health and wellness but there was the higher expectation to make the sale. That "just give them a quick intro and make the sale" mentality never really resonated with me. I was more concerned with providing as much of an education as I could. I was not aware of it at the time but these New Member Assessments gave me the opportunity to hone in on a template of introductory wellness education information, or the training-wheels of wellness, as I like to call it.

I had just wrapped up a New Member Assessment back in 2013 when I told myself "one of these days, I need to compile the training-wheels of wellness information I cover during these assessments into one place" and then that new member I just finished working with turned around and said "you know you should really put all of that information we covered into a book or something." Well after feeling dumbstruck, because I thought that member had just legitimately read my mind, I made a personal vow to put the information into a guide. After three years of "someday…" and using stick-figure cartoons as an artistic outlet, here it is.

This guide is intended to help individuals by providing a general overview of health and wellness from the insights of a Certified Personal Trainer. I use the training wheels of wellness information and approach with each new client I work with and experience excellent results. My goal with each client is to provide them with a solid foundation of information that covers three main topics associated with health (Eat, Train, & Rest). With the information found within these pages and continued dialogue, my clients are able to take off their metaphorical training wheels and navigate their health and wellness journey as informed students. Now, I would like to share the information with you!

The book is broken up into four parts (Reflect, Eat, Train, Rest) and is laid out in a way to provide information and help relate the information specifically to your life through some guided questions and reflections. It was my intention to deliver a lot of foundational principles associated with basic health and wellness in a fun way. You get to be the judge and I welcome questions and feedback via email!

THANK YOU AND ENJOY!

Email: tj@trainingwheelsofwellness.com

Welcome

Please answer these quick questions:

Question # 1

Have you ever thought to yourself or know someone to say something along the lines of "I wish I was healthier"?

YES   NO

If you answered "YES", get a pencil or some other sketching implement and keep reading. If you answered "NO", I would like to thank you for taking a break from your alternate universe to open this book/file and take a peak into our reality but why don't you go ahead and get back to enjoying your perfect genetic structure and utopia.

Question # 2

Do stick figures offend you?

YES   NO

If you answered "YES", please go talk through this issue with a trained professional and return when ready or maybe just donate this little gem to another person in your life. If you answered "NO", THANK YOU and ENJOY!

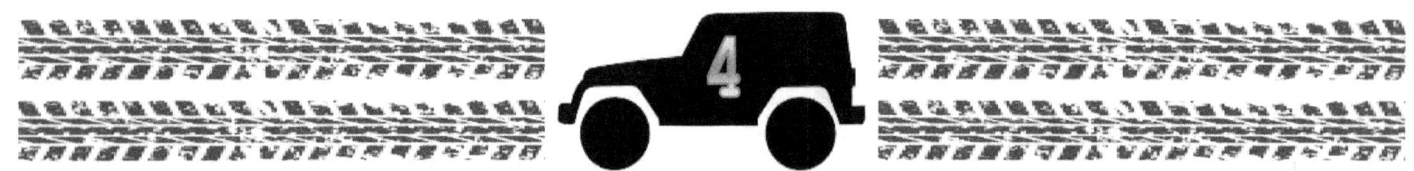

Greetings reader! I am TJ, well the stick-figure representation of TJ, and I will be your guide through this wonderful handbook. If you answered "YES" to question # 2 on the previous page, what are you doing here? Seriously, look at this face! How could I offend anyone? If you are reading this now, I guess you overcame your fear so just keep rolling with your newly found courage and keep up with the rest of us!

You may be asking yourself, "why a stick-figure?" and that's ok. I get it ALL the time. In the world of cartoon representation, the stick-figure is without a doubt the most versatile cartoon character that exists and probably more importantly, one of the easiest art forms to create.

So now that we met, let's move on to the fun! Oh and if you find yourself with questions, feel free to email me.

tj@trainingwheelsofwellness.com

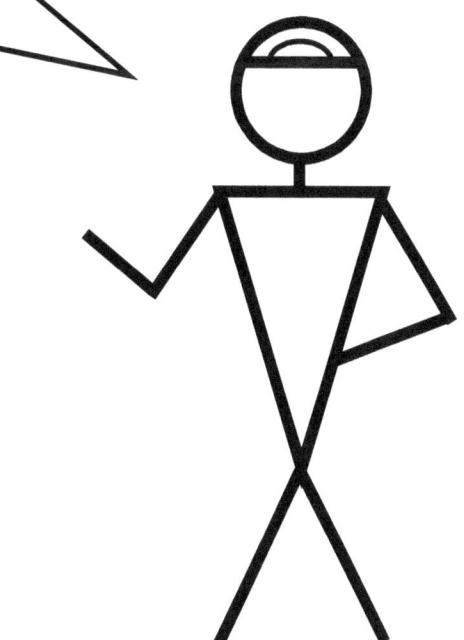

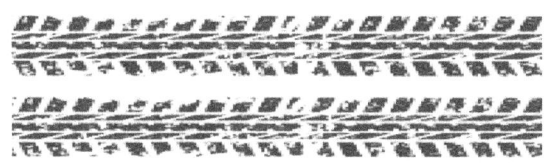  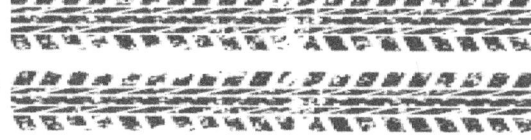

Today's date:

6 months:

12 months:

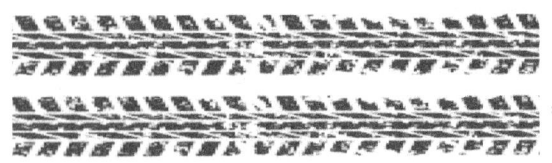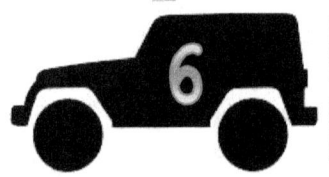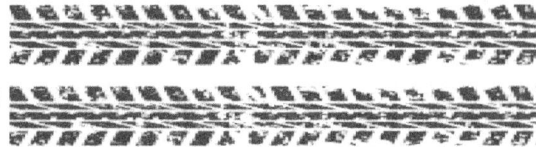

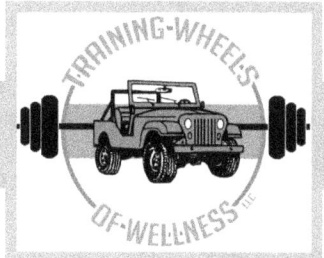

Part 1: Reflect

In this opening section, I am going to take you on a bit of a reflective journey. You owe it to yourself to answer questions and reflect with an honest heart.

The goal of this section is to help you recognize and accept your personal history, present situation, and hopeful future.

Once you are able to identify your personal reasons for wanting a change in your current situation for the sake of your future, you will have a very important tool at your disposal. These personal reasons become your motivational foundation. Whenever you are faced with the inevitable speedbumps that find their way into your life, you will be better equipped to overcome them and continue on your journey towards a healthier life.

It is also very important to share these reasons with trustworthy people in your life because they will help keep you accountable and remind you of your reasons and motivation for beginning the journey when the speedbumps get in your way. Trust me, it's awesome to have a team to help you during these moments.

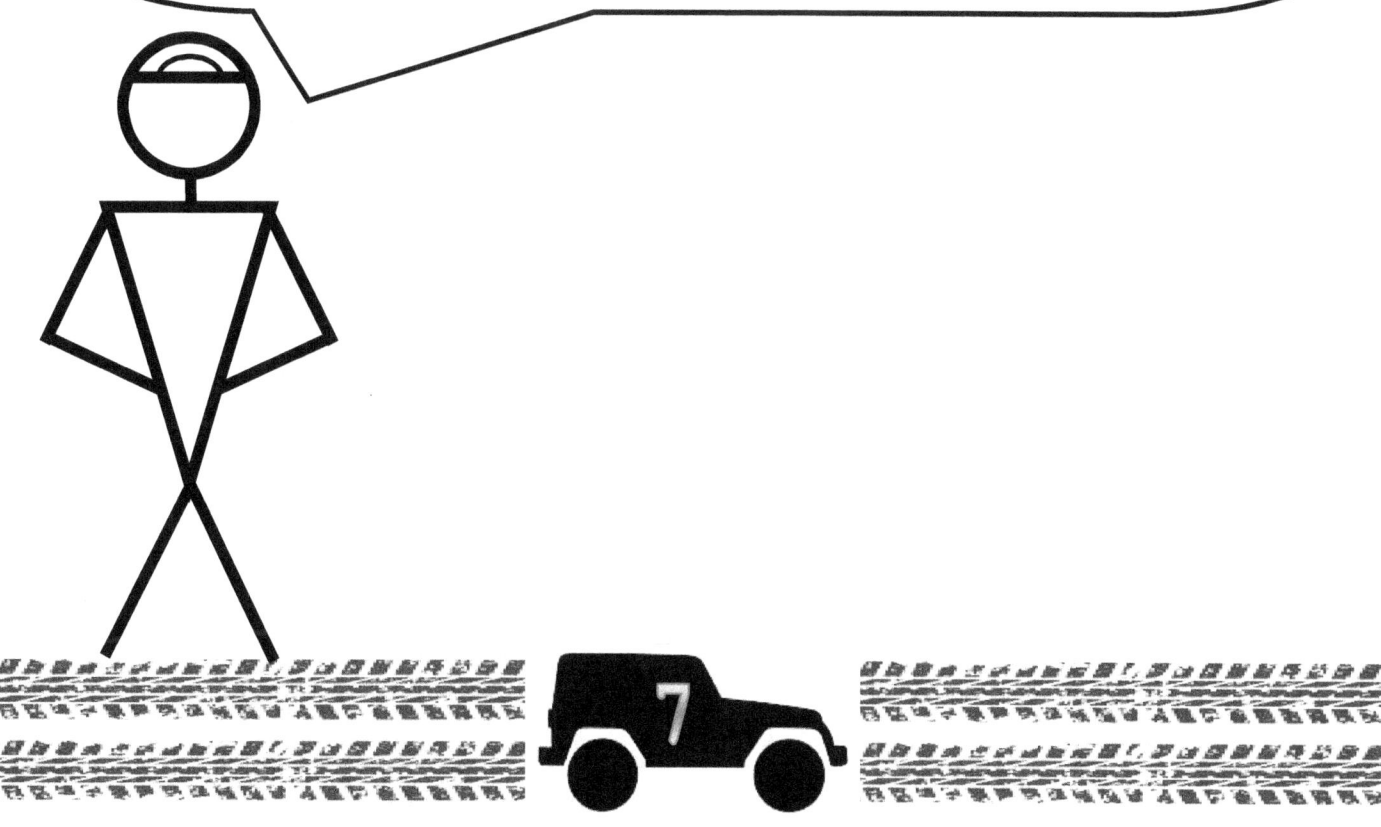

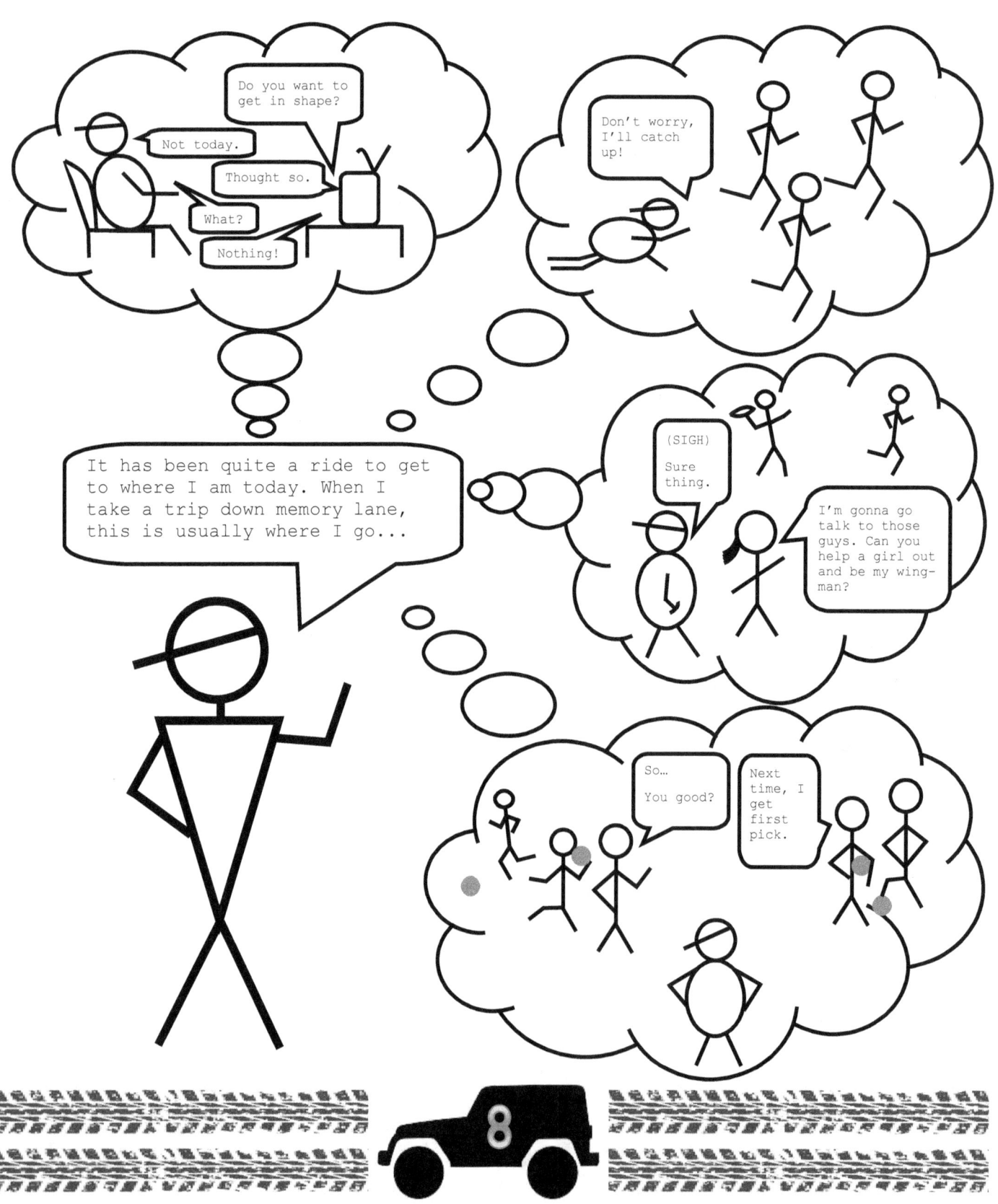

Take some time to write or sketch out some of your memories or current experiences that you consider to be motivation for your quest for wellness. Feel free to ask trusted people in your life for their input!

Potential Futures

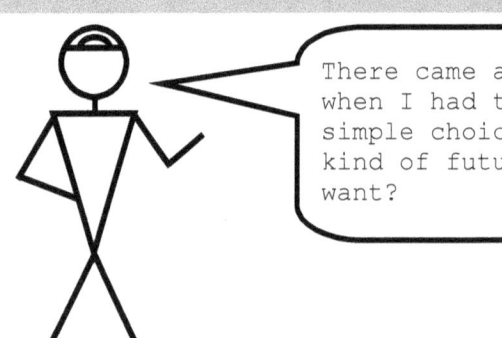

Scary Future VS Desired Future

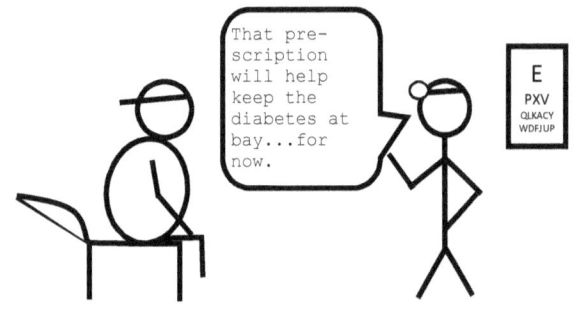
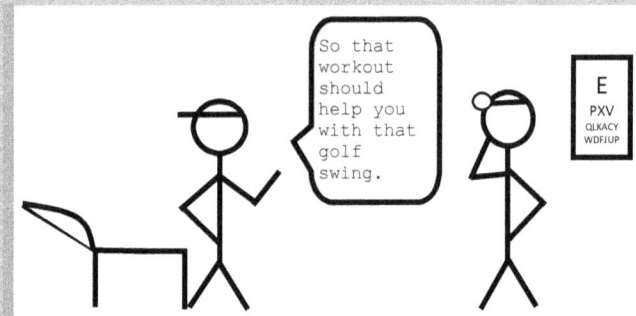

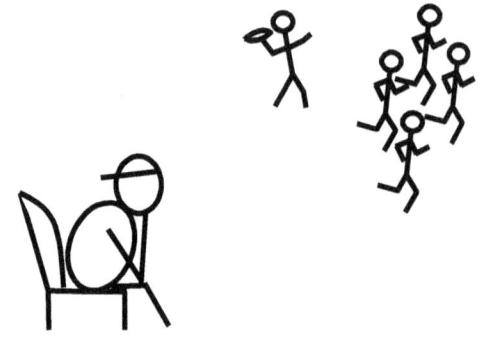
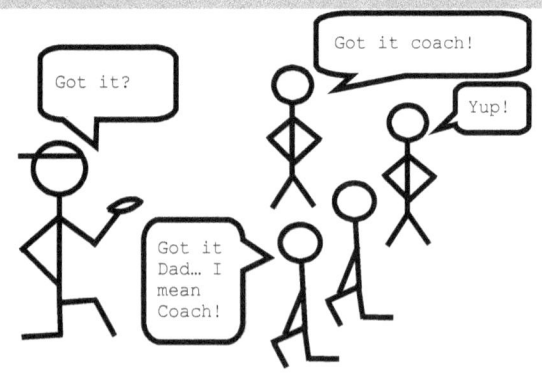

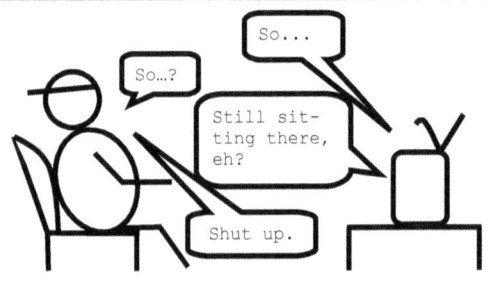
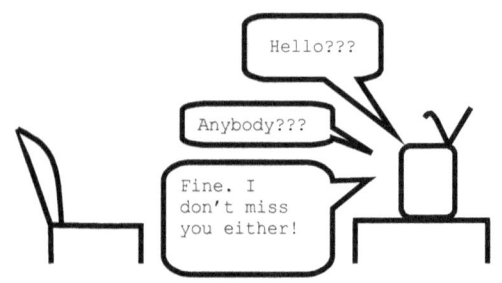

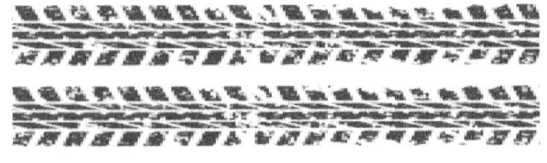
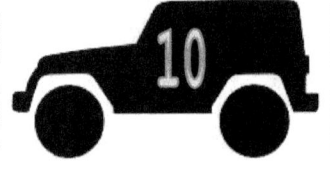

Scary Future 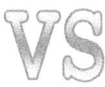 Desired Future

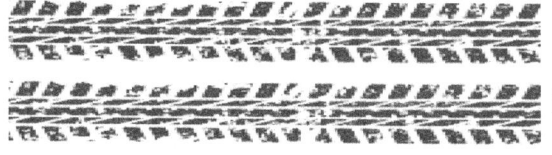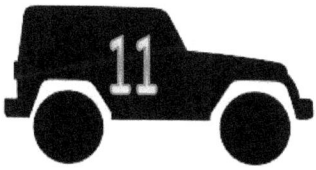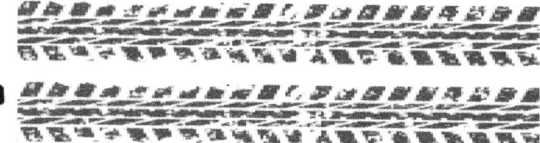

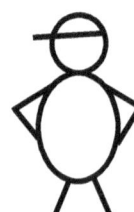

"After a few years of experimenting, this particular routine has helped me maintain the weight loss."

VS

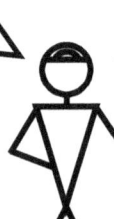

"We'll cover each topic in the following chapters to help you with your experiment."

Eat

• 3 - 4 meals/day	• 3 - 4 "built" meals/day
• Fast food 2 - 4 times/week	• 3 - 4 snacks/day
• 3 - 7 snacks/day	• Limited or no fast food, soda, or other sugary drinks
• 2 - 3 sugary drinks/day	• More whole foods, fewer processed foods
• Few fruits and veggies	

Train

• Sporadic recreational sports	• 3 total body workouts/week @30—45 minutes
• "Run? Why, is someone chasing me?"	• 3 run days/week @30—45 minutes
	• 1 LISS day/week

Rest

• 5 - 7 hours of sleep/night	• 7 - 8 hours of sleep/night
• 1 - 2 hour naps whenever time permitted	• 20 - 25 min siesta if needed after lunch
	• Alternate workout days with run days to rest the different muscle groups

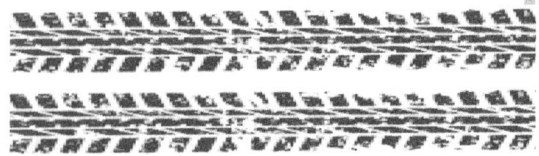

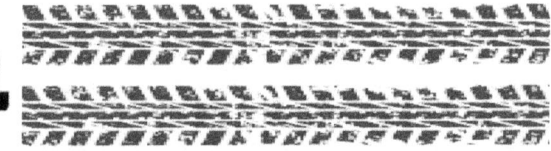

12

Your turn!

Current Behavior VS **Desired Behavior**

	Eat	
	Train	
	Rest	

The Wheel

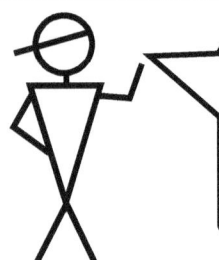

A good wheel needs to be balanced. This exercise illustrates how balanced your current approach to wellness is. Place your numbers accordingly and connect the dots as close to a circle as they allow. Once drawn, shade your circle in. If your wheel is out of balance, I suggest focusing in on the particular area that is throwing the wheel off balance before the others. A balanced approach to improved wellness will yield greater results.

Please identify your understanding and implementation of the topics below on the following scale of 1–10.

1 = I am THE worst

5–6 = I am alive, but not thriving with my current knowledge

10 = I should put this book down and go write my own on the topic

Eating: Nutrient & Calorie Consumption

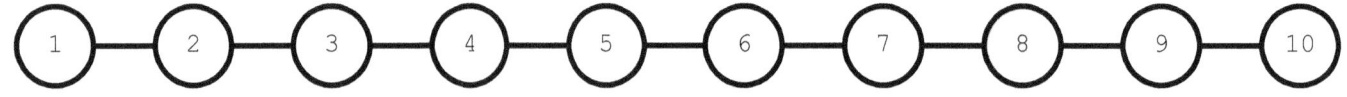

1 — 2 — 3 — 4 — 5 — 6 — 7 — 8 — 9 — 10

Training: Exercise Knowledge & Program Design

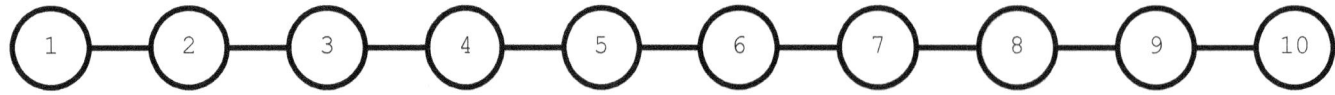

1 — 2 — 3 — 4 — 5 — 6 — 7 — 8 — 9 — 10

Resting: Active Rest & Sleeping Patterns

1 — 2 — 3 — 4 — 5 — 6 — 7 — 8 — 9 — 10

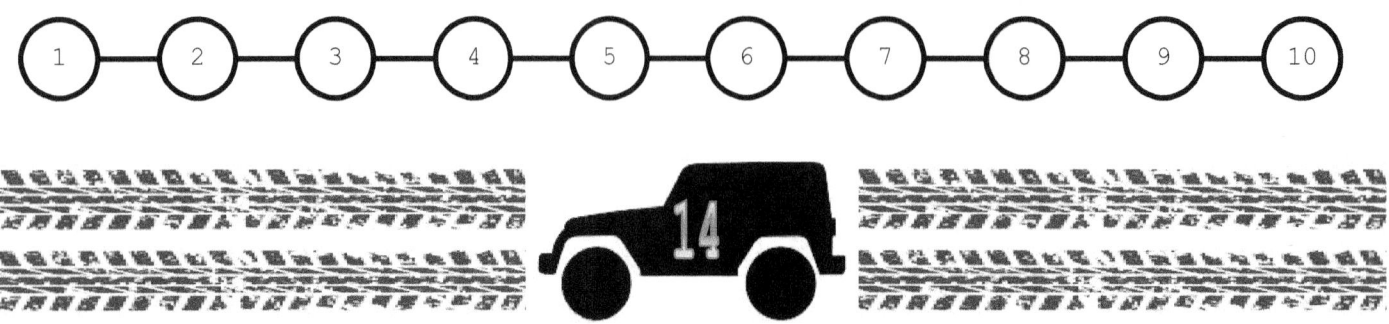

10

Training

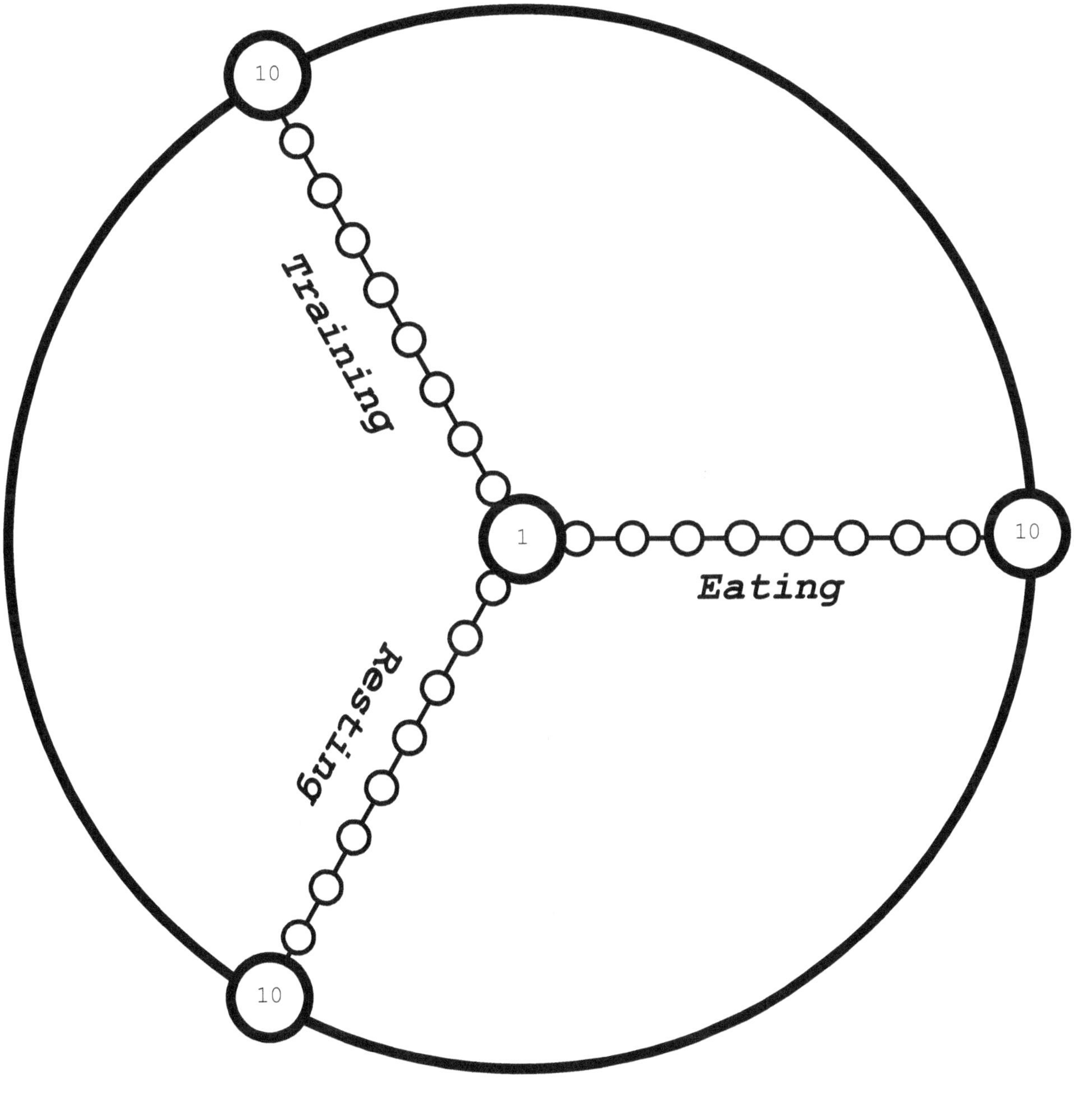

1

Eating

10

Resting

10

15

For further reflection and information:

- *https://www.nwmissouri.edu/wellness/PDF/shift/BalancingYourWellness.pdf*

- *https://www.macalester.edu/healthandwellness/sustainablestudent*

- *http://www.berkeleywellness.com/healthy-mind/mood/article/does-personality-affect-health*

- *https://und.edu/health-wellness/_files/docs/wellnessassessmentworksheet.pdf*

- *https://www3.uwrf.edu/Wellness*

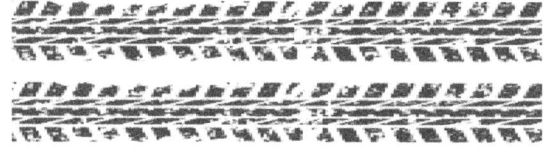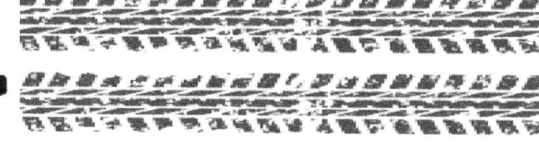

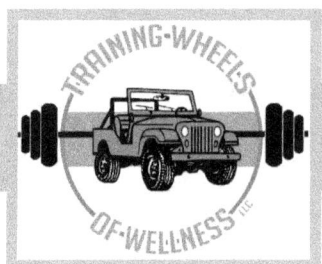

Part 2: Eat

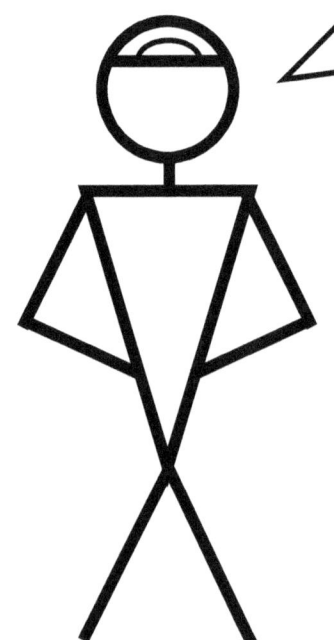

**DISCLAIMER: The following are basic nutrition guidelines. Please consult with your physician before beginning any new eating plan.

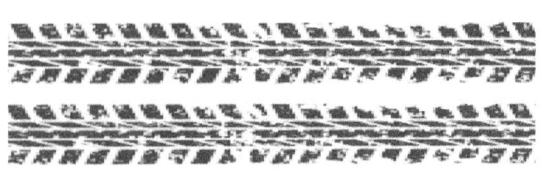

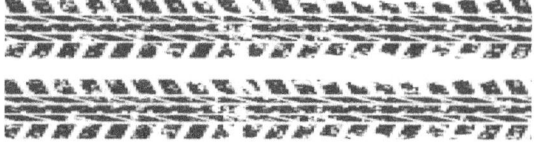

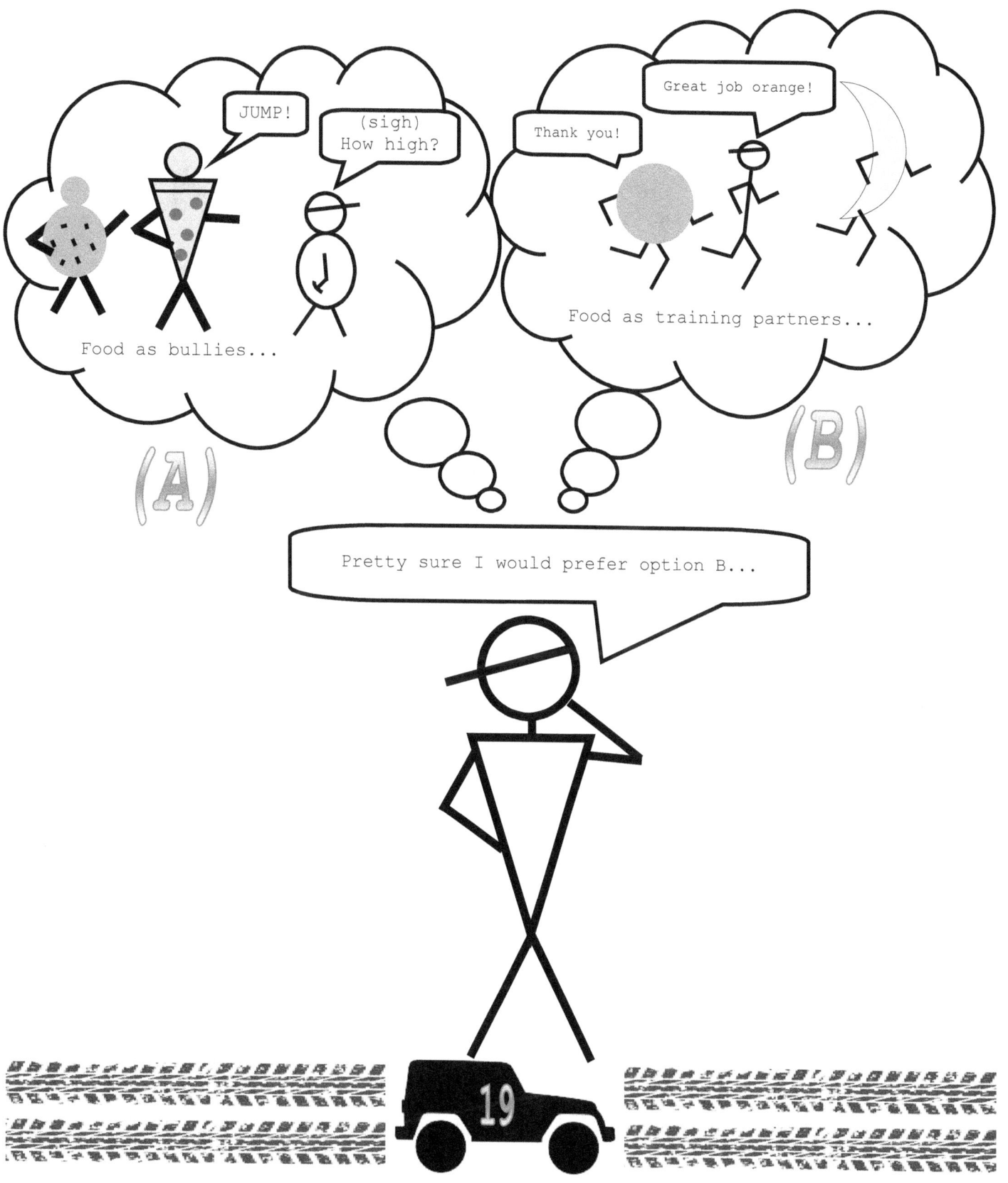

When most people begin a new diet, they tend to completely try and erase certain foods from their personal menu of options. This "all or nothing" approach is self-defeating. Diets that focus on eliminating certain foods lead to a sense of feeling powerless over oneself. The craving will build up over time until the "binge" happens which is when the individual over indulges in pleasure eating. The end result is a failed diet.

Instead of the strict "all or nothing" approach, I recommend developing a healthier relationship with food. A healthy relationship with food demonstrates a more consistent pattern of healthy consumption of healthy choices. So what does that look like? Well, for starters, internalize the following numbers suggested by many brilliant people for the proper ratio of the macro nutrients your body needs.

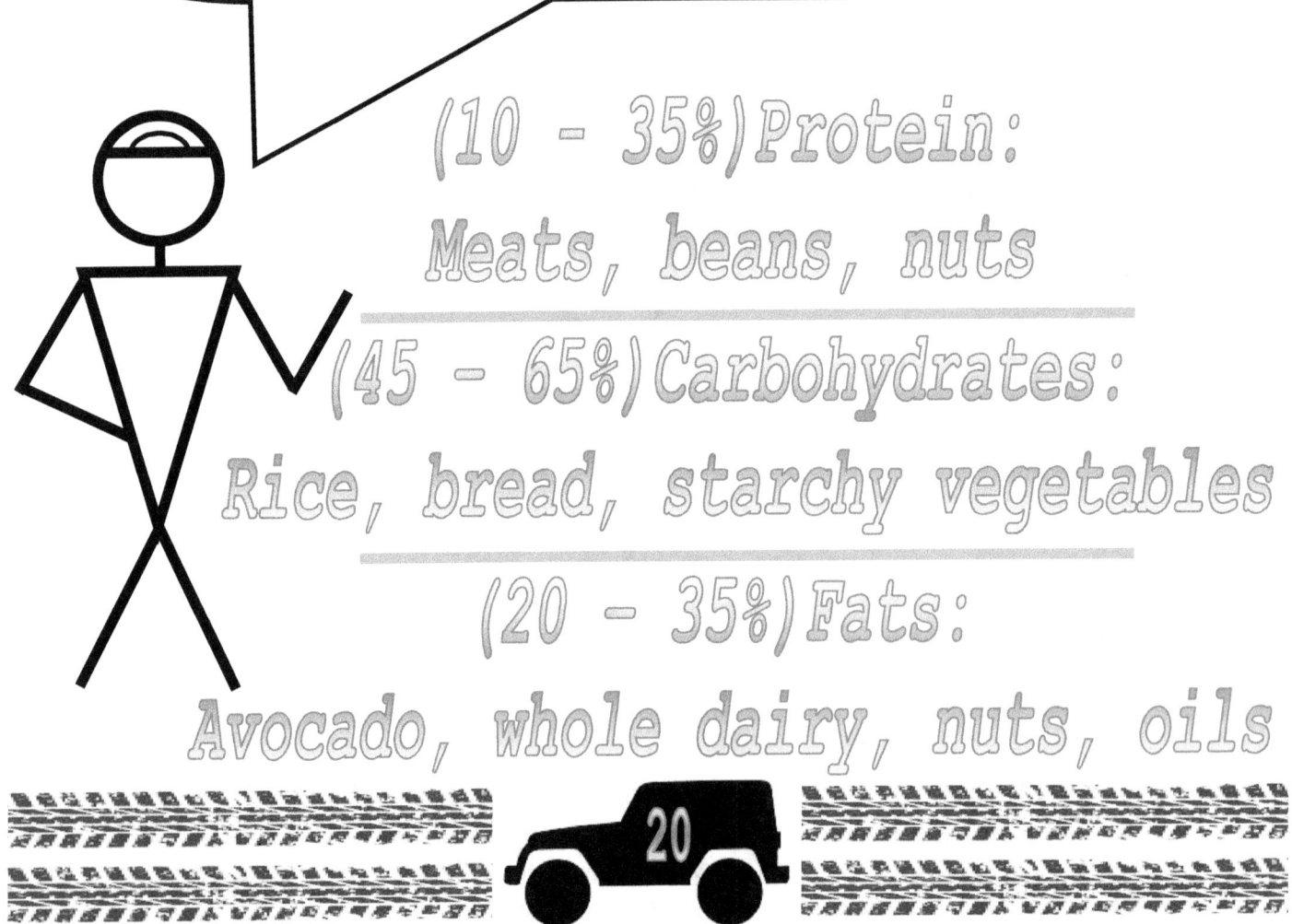

(10 - 35%) Protein:
Meats, beans, nuts

(45 - 65%) Carbohydrates:
Rice, bread, starchy vegetables

(20 - 35%) Fats:
Avocado, whole dairy, nuts, oils

20

I have no shame in letting you know that chocolate chip cookies are my BIGGEST weakness… I am human. Before we get to the calorie math fun, I wanted to point out the sugar and sodium content found on nutrition labels. Be very mindful of your sugar and sodium intakes. Processed foods are notorious for having high levels of both and over time, can lead to health concerns.

Chocolate Chip

Nutrition Facts

Serving size 1 cookie (40g)

Calories 150	Fat Calories 50	
		% Daily Value*
Total Fat 5g		7%
Saturated 3g		15%
Trans 0g		
Cholesterol 15mg		7%
Sodium 80mg		3%
Total Carbs 19g		6%
Dietary Fiber 4g		16%
Sugars 9g		
Protein 10g		20%

Vitamin A 0%	•	Vitamin C	40%
Calcium 15%	•	Iron	1%

*Percent Daily Values (DV) are based on a 2,000 calorie diet.

Ingredients:

Hormone-Free Whey and Milk Protein Concentrates (rBST/rBGH-free), Chocolate Chips (Sugar, Chocolate Liquor, Cocoa Butter, Vanilla), Organic Brown Rice Syrup, Organic Inulin (Blue Agave), Vegetable Glycerin, Brown Sugar, Organic Coconut Oil, Sunflower Oil, Filtered Water, Natural Flavors, Non-GMO Sunflower Lecithin, Baking Soda, Sea Salt, Antioxidant Blend (Decaffeinated Green Tea Extract, Vit C (ascorbic acid)), Stevia Leaf Extract (Natural Sweetener), and Xanthan Gum Non-GMO all natural ingredients.

Contains Milk. Manufactured in a Facility that Processes Peanuts, Eggs, Treenuts, Soy and Wheat.

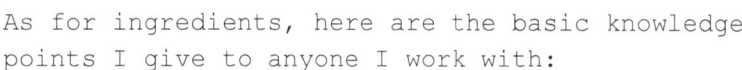

As for ingredients, here are the basic knowledge points I give to anyone I work with:

- Ingredients are listed in order of their contribution to the finished food product. For example, the first ingredient listed makes up the most of the finished food item.

- Whenever you can, I highly recommend the purchase of food items that you are able to pronounce the ingredients found within them. Basically, if you are not able to pronounce the ingredients, think twice about what is going into your body.

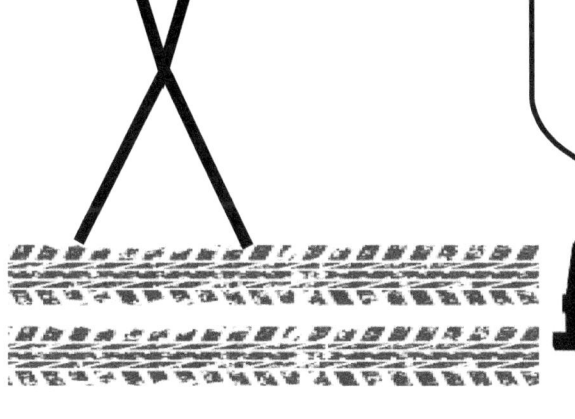

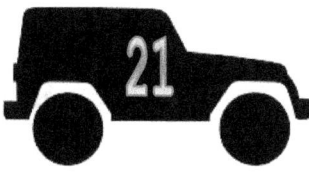

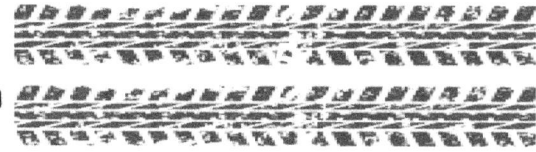

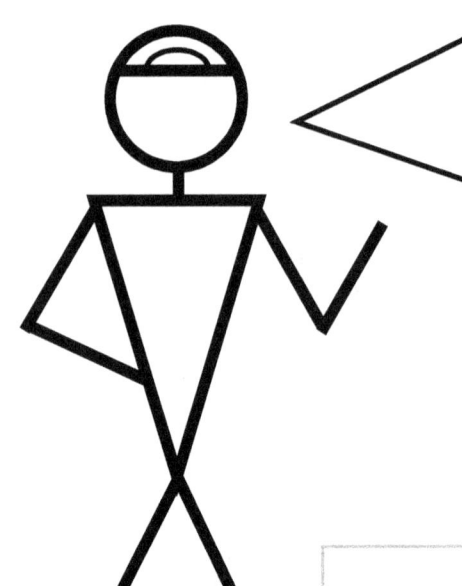

Ok so please try and contain your excitement for this next activity… You ok? You sure? Ready? Ok...time for some MATH! WOOOOO!!!

The chart below illustrates how to find the amount of calories derived from the macronutrients in a food. Most food labels will give you the grams found in the food.

For the example below, there are 6 grams of protein found in an average egg. In order to figure out how many calories from protein, multiply the number of grams by 4. Out of the 69 total calories found in an egg, 24 calories come from protein. The remaining 45 calories come from fat (5 grams X 9 = 45).

Macronutrient	Protein	Carbohydrates	Fats
Calories/Gram	4	4	9
Example: Egg	6 grams = 24 calories	0	5 grams = 45 calories
Total Calories (1 large egg)	69 calories (24 protein + 45 fat)		

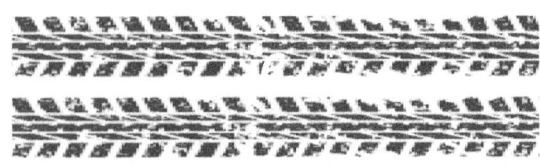 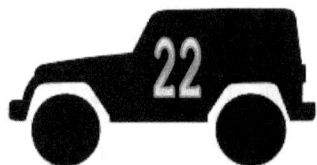 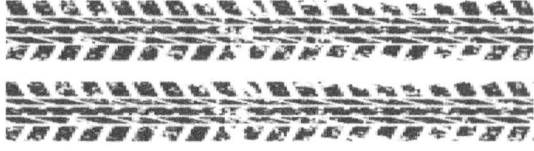

Now let's take the egg example and use it in a "built" meal. A "built" meal includes all of the macronutrients and the nutrients are properly represented to reflect the recommended percentage of caloric intake.

In the chart below you will find that this particular meal represents the macronutrients as follows:

Carbohydrates: 50%; Protein: 19%; Fat; 31%

These percentages fall within the healthy ranges recommended by the Food and Drug Administration.

Throughout the day, I recommend three "built" meals supplemented by healthy snacks. Check out how your numbers add up on the next page then compare a healthy day with a "cheat" day.

Built Meal Example

Ingredient	Calories	Carbohy-drate Calories	Protein Calories	Fat Calories
2 Eggs	138	0	48	90
Whole Wheat Toast (2	136	98	19	19
Spinach (1 cup)	8	4	4	0
Hummus Spread (2tbspn)	50	16	8	26
Salsa (2 servings)	70	56	14	0
Corn Tortilla Chips (1 serving)	120	85	8	27
Totals	522	259	101	162
Percentages	100%	50%	19%	31%

Daily Intake

Food or Drink Item	Calories	Carbohydrate Calories	Protein Calories	Fat Calories
Totals				
Percentages	100%			

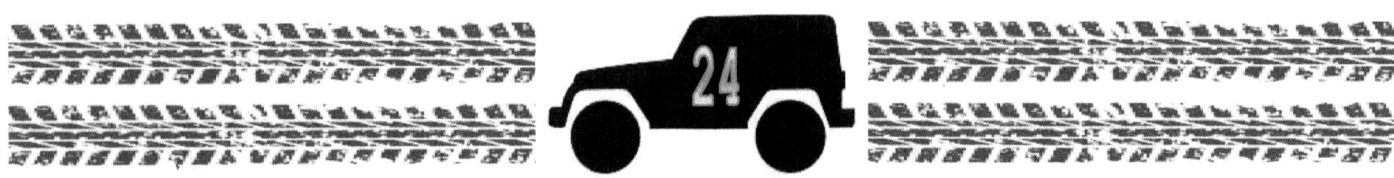

Daily Intake

Food or Drink Item	Calories	Carbohydrate Calories	Protein Calories	Fat Calories
Totals				
Percentages	100%			

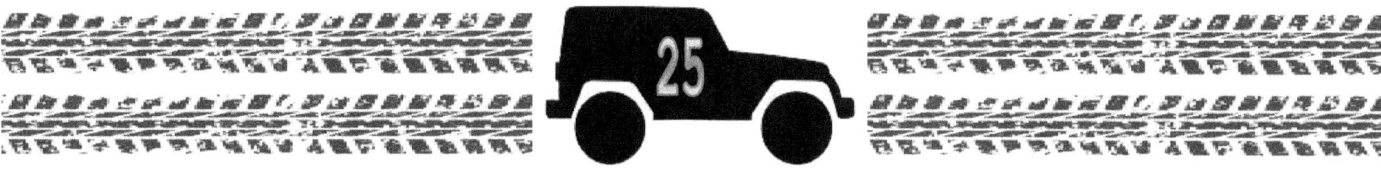

For further reflection and information:

- *http://www.whfoods.com/foodstoc.php*

- *http://www.fda.gov/Food/default.htm*

- *http://www.huffingtonpost.com/entry/healthiest-diets-world_us_57cc716fe4b0a22de0966ff2*

- *ANY book by Michael Pollan: http://michaelpollan.com*

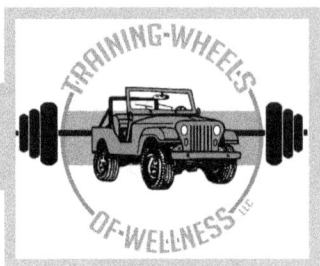

Part 3: Train

We're going to cover a lot of ground in this section. Basically, we're going to go back to basics and learn how to combine basic exercises into fun circuits that can help you accomplish a new body-type.

I will also give you some tips and rules for guidance and to help lower the chance of common injuries often experienced by beginners.

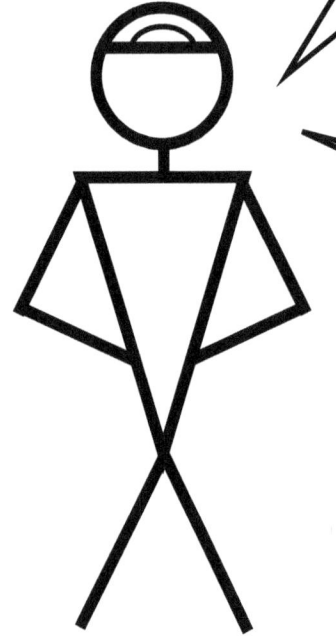

**DISCLAIMER: The following are basic fitness guidelines. Please consult with your physician before beginning any new fitness plan.

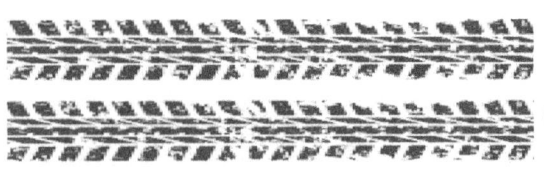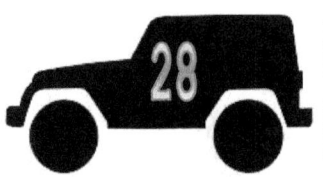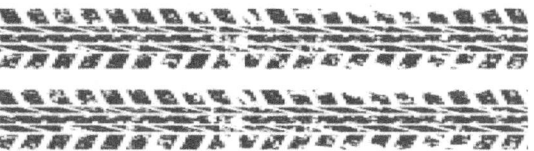

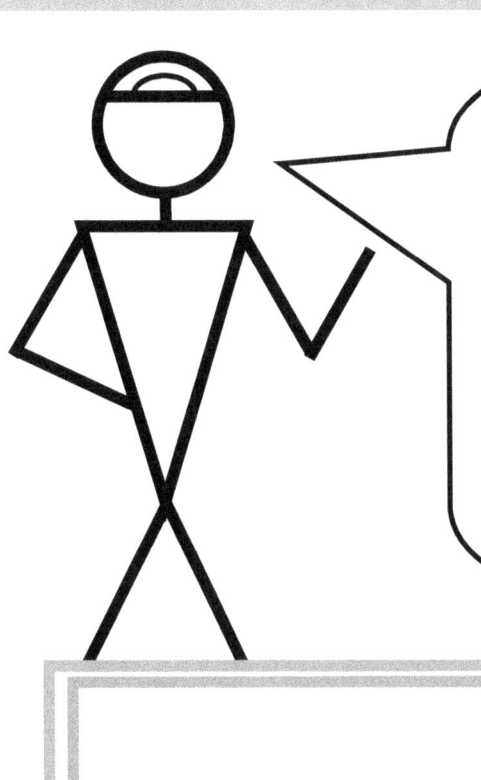

This is the topic that as a trainer, I am supposed to present some amazing new formula or recipe for success that incorporates miraculous exercises that enhance muscle development.

Sorry...not going to happen.

Before moving into the advanced movements that the body is capable of, it is VITAL to establish a foundation of confidence with the basic movements that are time-tested and PROVEN to work.

In the following pages, we'll cover the movements that help establish your chest, back, legs, and core from which many other exercises are derived.

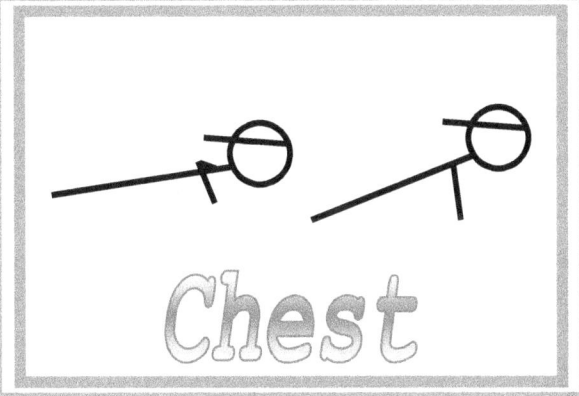

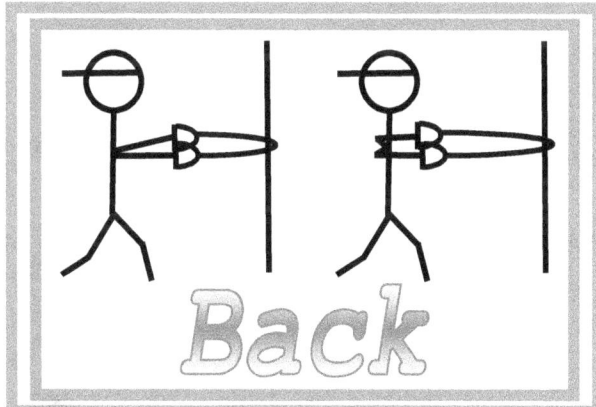

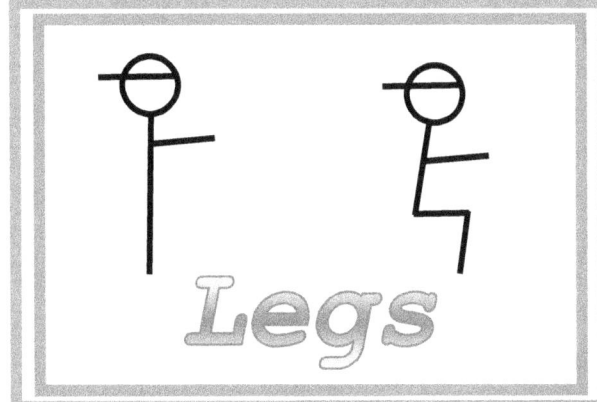

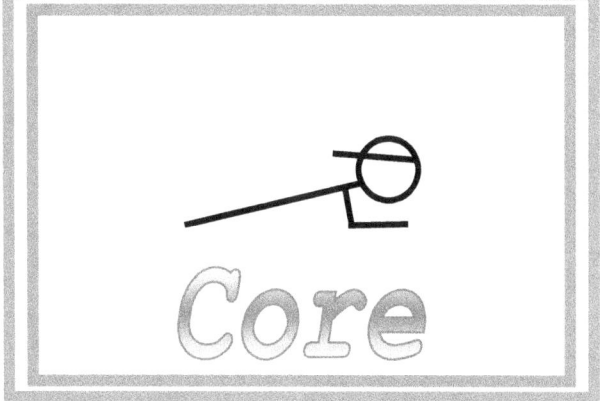

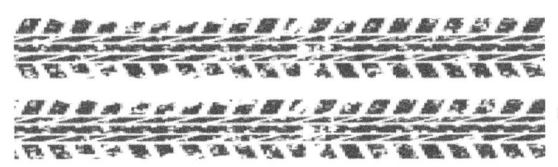

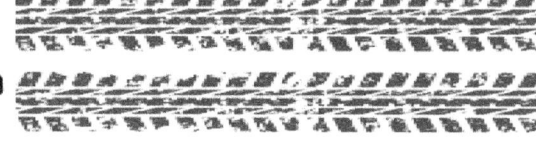

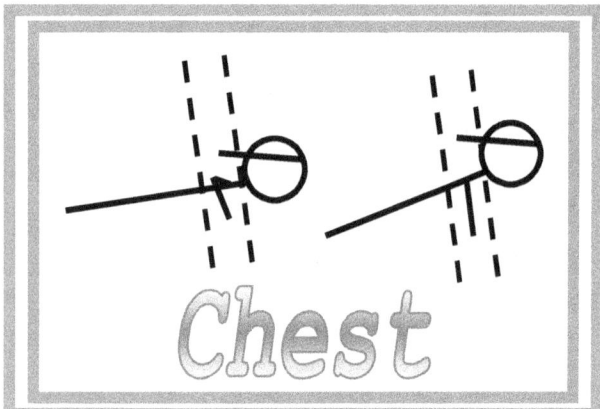

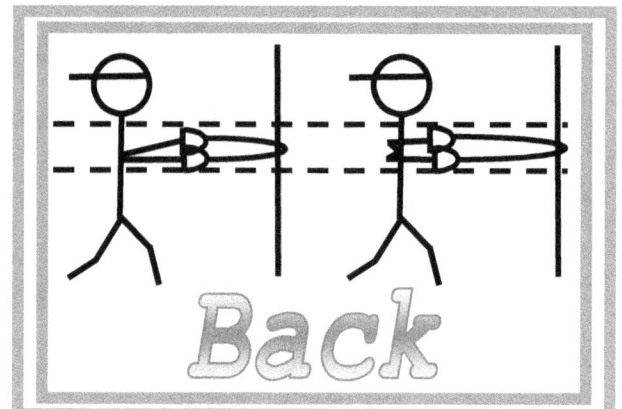

The hand-heart-hand rule: Whenever performing a push or pull-type exercise, keep your hands and elbows in line with your heart rather than way up high towards the shoulders.

Hand   Heart   Hand

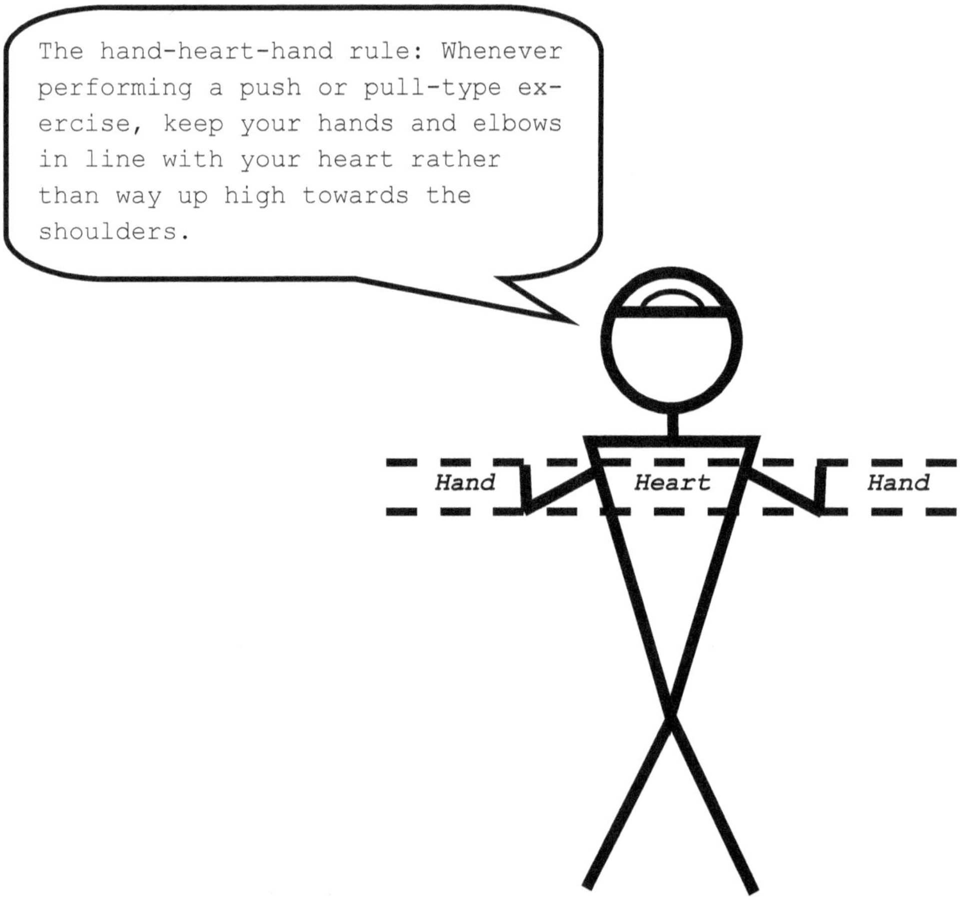

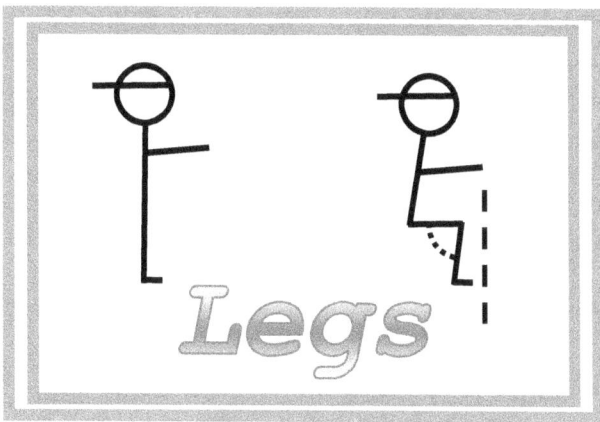

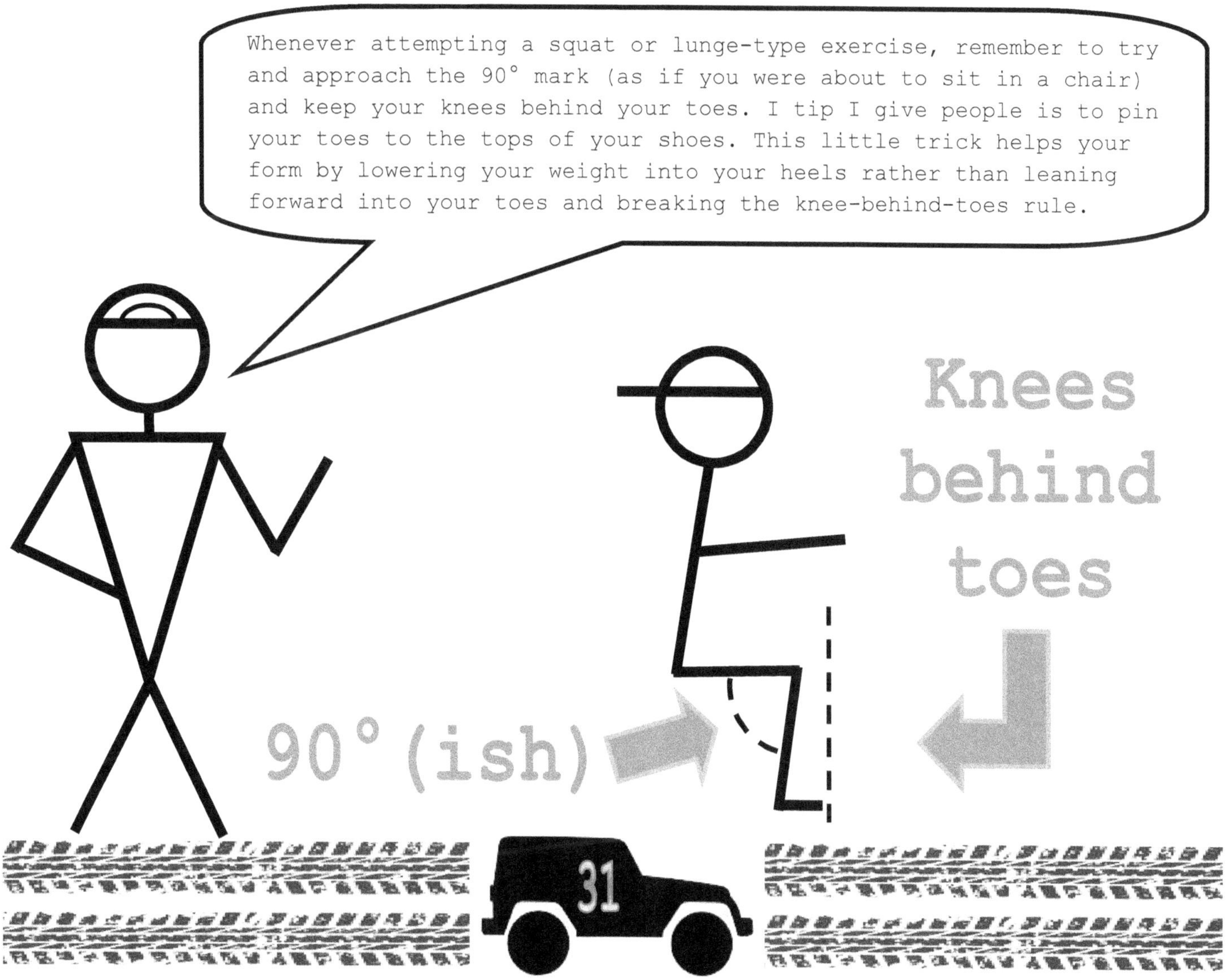

Whenever attempting a squat or lunge-type exercise, remember to try and approach the 90° mark (as if you were about to sit in a chair) and keep your knees behind your toes. I tip I give people is to pin your toes to the tops of your shoes. This little trick helps your form by lowering your weight into your heels rather than leaning forward into your toes and breaking the knee-behind-toes rule.

Knees
behind
toes

90°(ish)

31

Proper breathing, like proper form, is VITAL to a successful workout. Below are the breathing patterns you should use while performing various exercises. The basic rule I share with everyone I work with is to BREATHE OUT whenever you are moving AGAINST gravity or using force to move an object and BREATHE IN as you reset. You are more likely to maintain control over your heartrate if you are able to control your breathing.

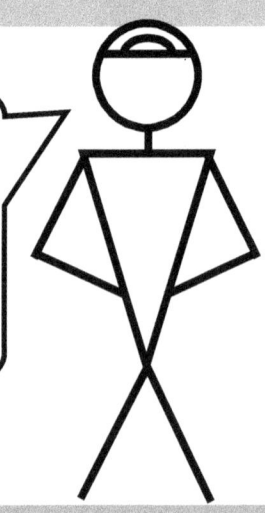

Chest

Inhale a breath as you lower yourself

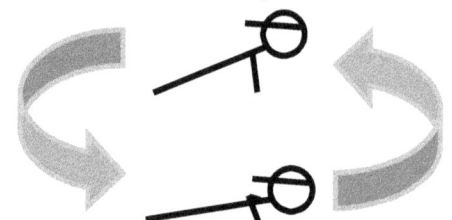

Exhale as you push yourself back up to the starting position

Back

Exhale as you perform the pull motion

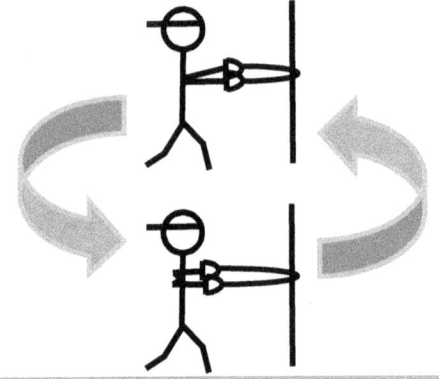

Inhale again as you return back to the starting position

Legs

Inhale a breath as you lower yourself

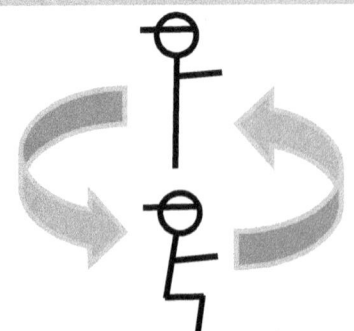

Exhale as you push yourself back up to the starting position

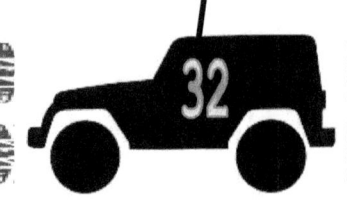

Did you ever play with Silly Putty as a kid? That stuff is amazing. It can stretch, be molded, and even copy comics from a newspaper! I like to use it now as a metaphor for muscle stretching.

If you stretch Silly Putty quickly and without warming it up, it will snap into two pieces. For muscles...that is NOT ideal. If you roll that Silly Putty gently in your hands for a little while, it will stretch and stretch and stretch for ages.

I suggest moving around with an activity such as jumping rope, jumping jacks, or simple calisthenics or yoga to increase blood flow to the muscles before stretching them.

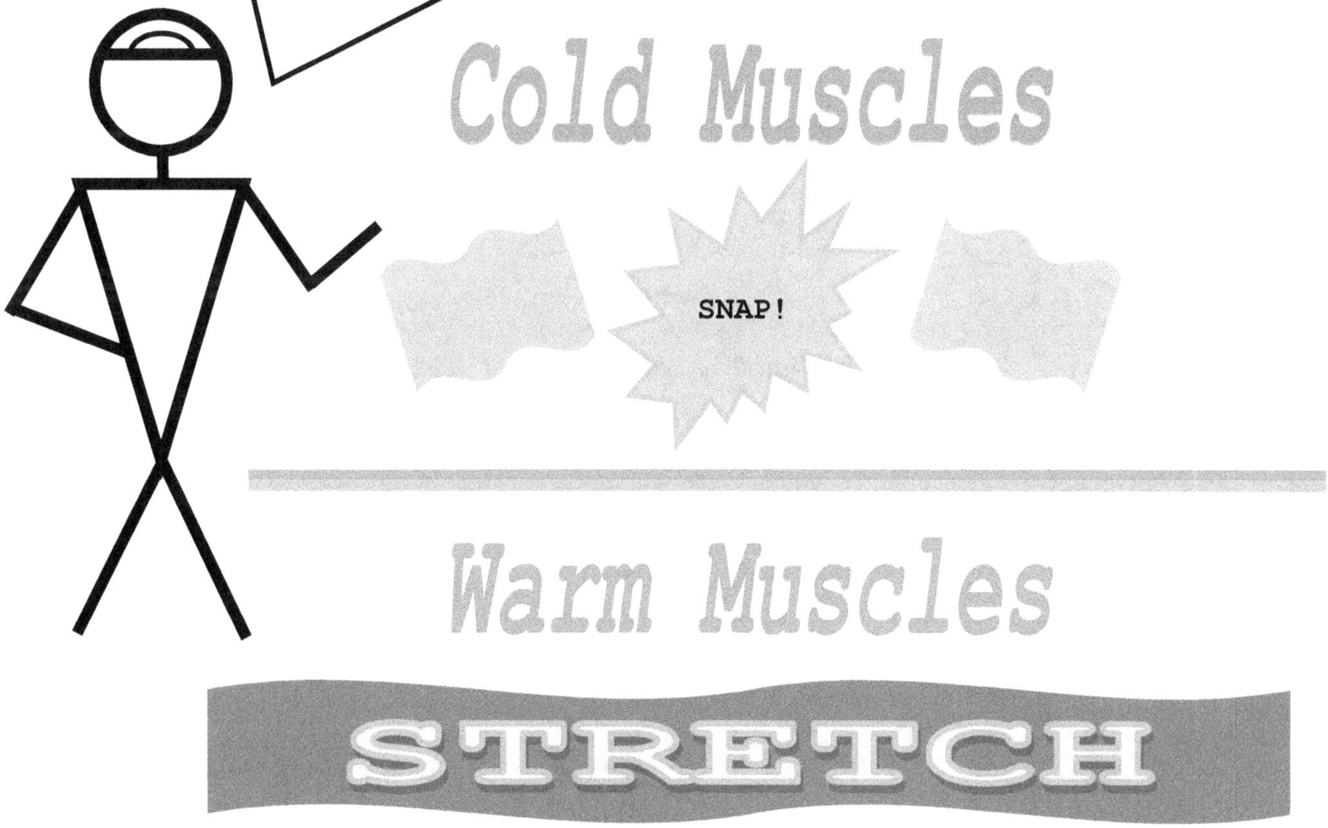

Cold Muscles

SNAP!

Warm Muscles

STRETCH

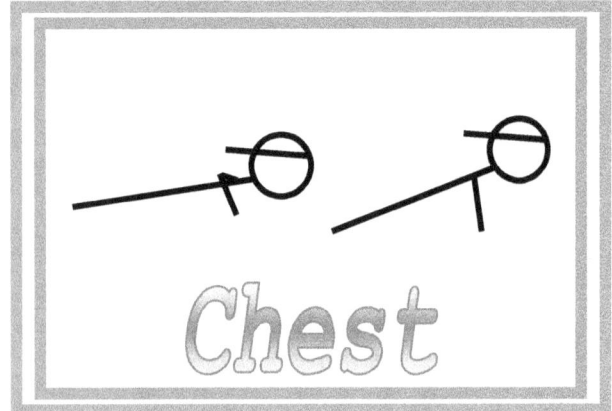

The Breathing Reminder:

Inhale a breath as you lower yourself

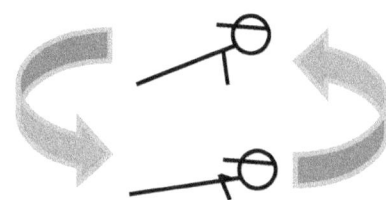

Exhale as you push yourself back up to the starting position

The Move: Pushup

The push-up is an example of a chest press and is such an amazing exercise that requires more muscles than people think. The primary muscle used to perform the pushup is the chest but the arms, core, and back are also recruited to assist the chest throughout the movement.

Start in the standard pushup position and while following the hand-heart-hand rule, lower yourself until your elbows are bent at approximately a 90° angle then return to the starting position.

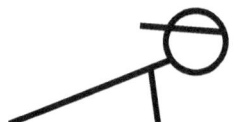  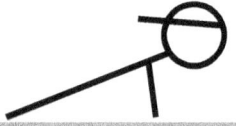

The Progression: Change the angle; change the difficulty!

Many individuals I work with for the first time cannot do a standard push-up on the ground and that is perfectly ok. The pushup can be modified. I tell folks to bring the floor closer to them by using an elevated surface like a park bench, sturdy chair, SUV bumper, Smith Machine (found in many gyms), or even the wall. Over time, you can change the angle to progress towards standard pushups then on to incline pushups which are even more challenging.

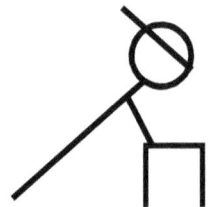 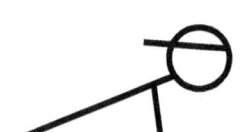 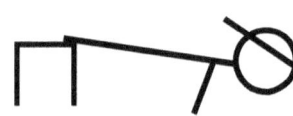

Beginner   **Intermediate**   **Advanced**

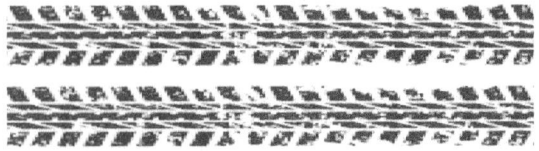 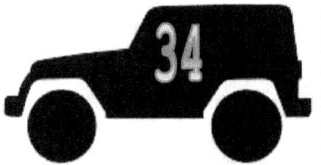 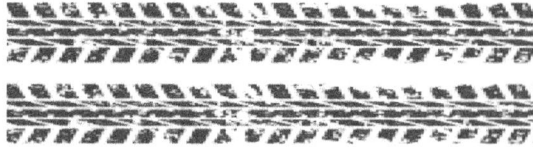

The Breathing Reminder:

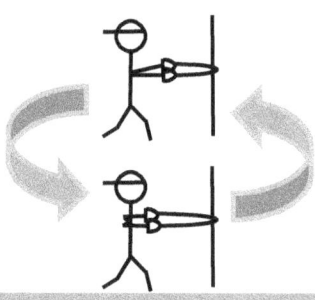

Exhale as you perform the pull motion

Inhale again as you return back to the starting position

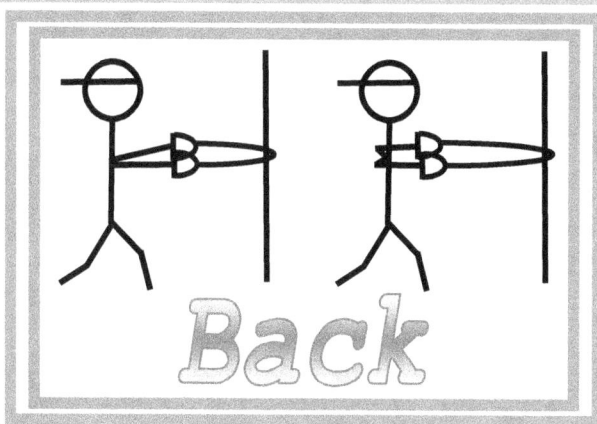

The Move: Back Rows

Whenever I work with someone new to fitness and wellness, I recommend the back row exercise as a great entry-level exercise that can help prepare the back muscles for eventual pull-up training. The back row exercise can be performed in a variety of ways by using different forms of resistance. Below, the resistance is provided by a rubber resistance band.

Begin this exercise with relaxed shoulders and keep the handles in line with the hand-heart-hand rule. Perform the pull motion by squeezing the shoulder blades together (as if someone was holding a marker in between your shoulder blades and you are trying to grasp it between your shoulder blades) and using your arms to assist. While performing the motion, keep your shoulders relaxed rather than shrugging up towards your neck and plant your feet in an A-frame as demonstrated below.

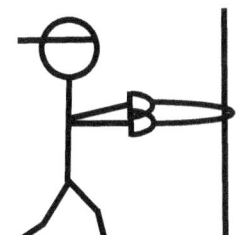 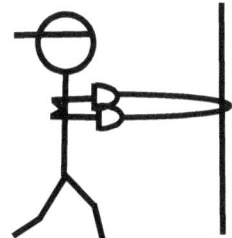 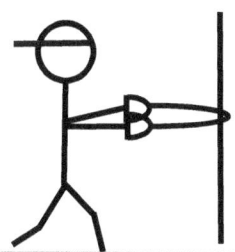

The Progression: Add resistance for bulk or reps for endurance

Depending on the body-type you are looking to emulate, you can add weight/resistance to build up muscle mass or add reps to start increasing muscle endurance without adding the bulk.

This exercise can also help prepare the muscles required for pull-up training which is a phenomenal back exercise for intermediate and advanced training.

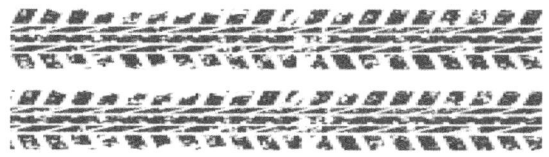 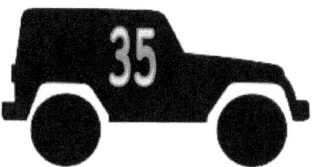 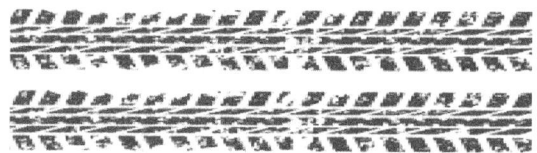

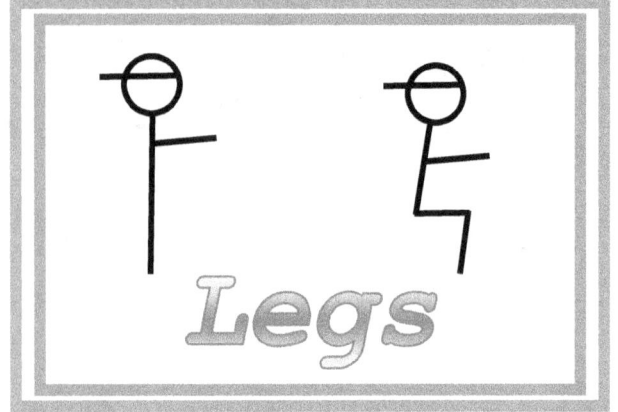

Legs

The Breathing Reminder:

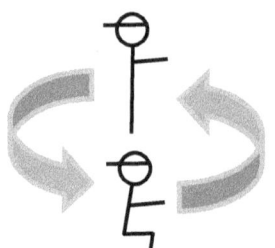

Inhale a breath as you lower yourself

Exhale as you push yourself back up to the starting position

The Move: Squats

In my opinion, the basic bodyweight squat is an underrated exercise that deserves to be implemented more often. To perform a proper squat, the body recruits the entire leg as well as the glutes (butt). Trainers are also trained to use the squat exercise as a means to demonstrate muscle readiness in prospective clients. Basically, this exercise can help us trainers as an indicator as to how fit an individual already is...or is not.

To perform a proper squat, use the 90°(ish) and toes-behind-the-knee rule and pretend to sit down in a chair, inhaling as you lower. Exhale as you push yourself back up to the beginning position. You may use your arms to reach out for balance.

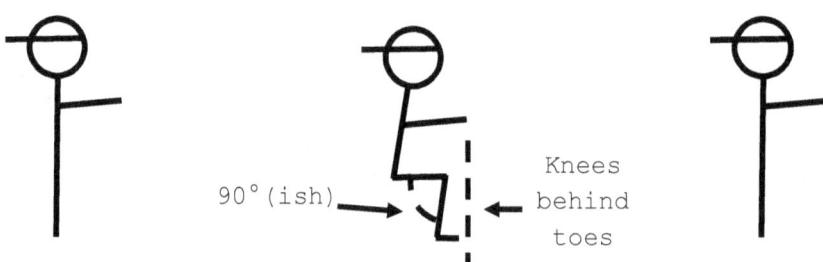

90°(ish)

Knees behind toes

The Progression: Add resistance for bulk or reps for endurance

Depending on the body-type you are looking to emulate, you can add weight/resistance to build up muscle mass or add reps to start increasing muscle endurance without adding the bulk.

This exercise can also be used for power training by jumping up and landing back in squat position or as a compound exercise that includes a secondary movement like a shoulder press.

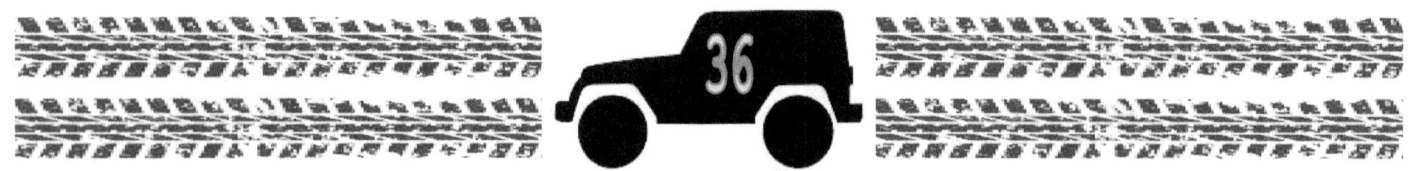

The Breathing Reminder:

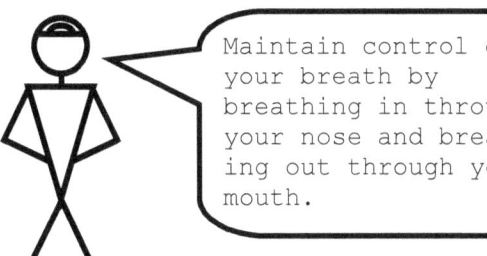

Maintain control of your breath by breathing in through your nose and breathing out through your mouth.

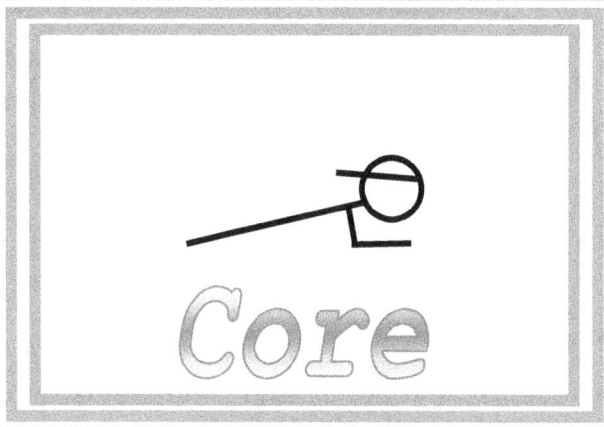

Core

The Move: Plank

The plank is a great exercise to start out with because of its simplicity and effectiveness. This exercise requires the entire body to do some work and with practice, you will see obvious results in terms of the amount of time you can hold the position.

To perform a proper plank, keep your body in a rigid line from your heels to the base of your neck. Instead of the hand-heart-hand rule, follow the elbow-heart-elbow rule to keep your weight dispersed properly over your elbows which will also protect your shoulders from unnecessary strain. You could follow the hand-heart-hand rule if you decide to try planking in the standard pushup position.

Similar to pushups, the angle decides the resistance.

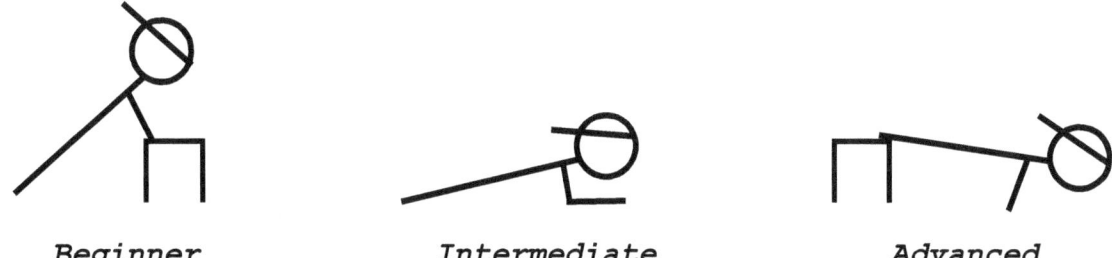

| Beginner | Intermediate | Advanced |

The Progression: Change the angle; change the difficulty and then add time

Aside from changing the angle, you can also try using unstable surfaces like a bosu-ball or stability ball which are commonly found in gyms. Before advancing to these unstable surfaces, I do recommend picking a plank position and challenge you to increase your time by practicing that same position for a while. Try for 30 seconds, then for 45 seconds, and keep trying for more as your workouts progress. The goal is to advance your time as often as you add reps and sets to other exercises in your workout.

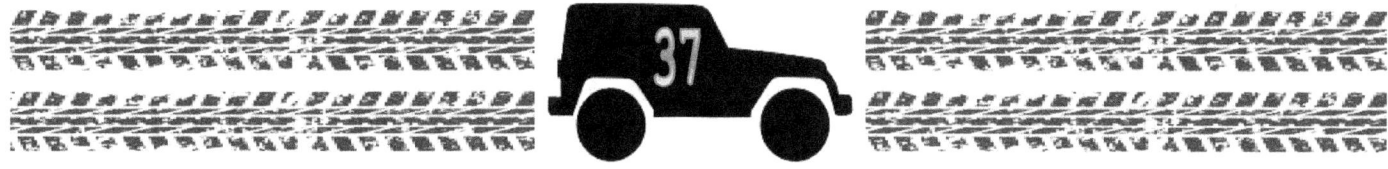

Circuit training is a wonderful way to experience the benefits that both strength and cardiovascular training have to offer. Cardiovascular benefits are able to be obtained when a set of strength training exercises are performed in an order with limited rest in between exercises. As one muscle group rests, another muscle group goes to work.

On the right, you will find an example of a simple circuit. Individually, each of these exercises targets a major muscle group but when combined into a circuit, these exercises form a total body workout. Here is an example of a quick circuit:

- Exercise 1: Pushups
- 30-60 seconds rest
- Exercise 2: Back rows
- 30-60 seconds rest
- Exercise 3: Bodyweight squats
- 30-60 seconds rest
- Exercise 4: Plank
- Water break (Less than 3 minutes)
- Repeat for 2 or 3 sets (20-30 min)

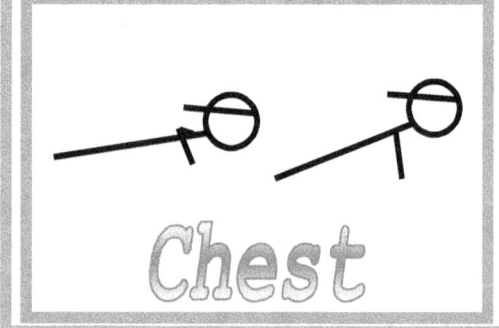

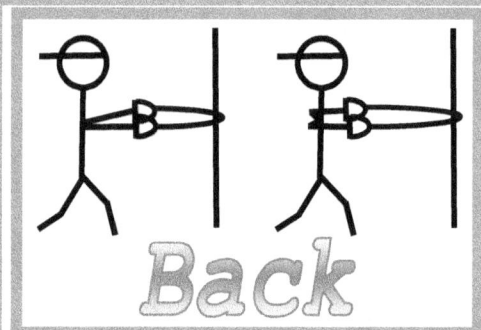

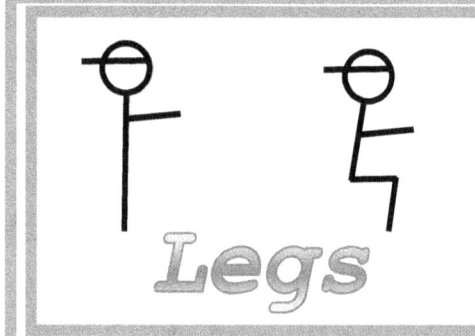

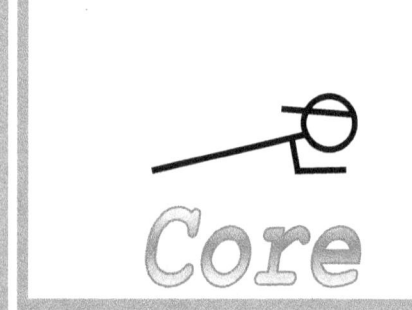

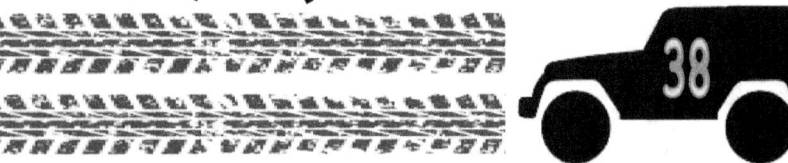

On the next two pages, you will find a menu of exercise options to choose from. There are many other exercises in the fitness world that could be added to the menu but it was my intention to keep it simple for the sake of providing you with a simple overview of building a circuit from a simple menu.

The Basic Circuit presented on the previous page has one exercise selected for each major muscle group. To build a larger circuit, simply add an exercise from the following menu for each muscle group. Instead of completing 4 exercises, you will be completing 8 exercises for your workout as you progress from a beginner to novice.

For your next progression from novice to experienced, add another exercise for each muscle group for a total of 12 exercises in your circuit.

By now you are probably asking yourself "how many rounds or sets of the circuit should I do?" and that is an excellent question!

Beginners: Aim for 2 sets of any new circuit

Intermediate: Aim for 3 sets

Advanced: 3 sets plus added repetitions or resistance/exercise

As for repetitions and resistance, choose a resistance that you are **safely** able to complete the chosen number of repetitions with. If your form starts to suffer, choose a different resistance or number of repetitions.

If you google any of the exercises listed on the menu, you will be able to find an instructional video how to perform them properly.

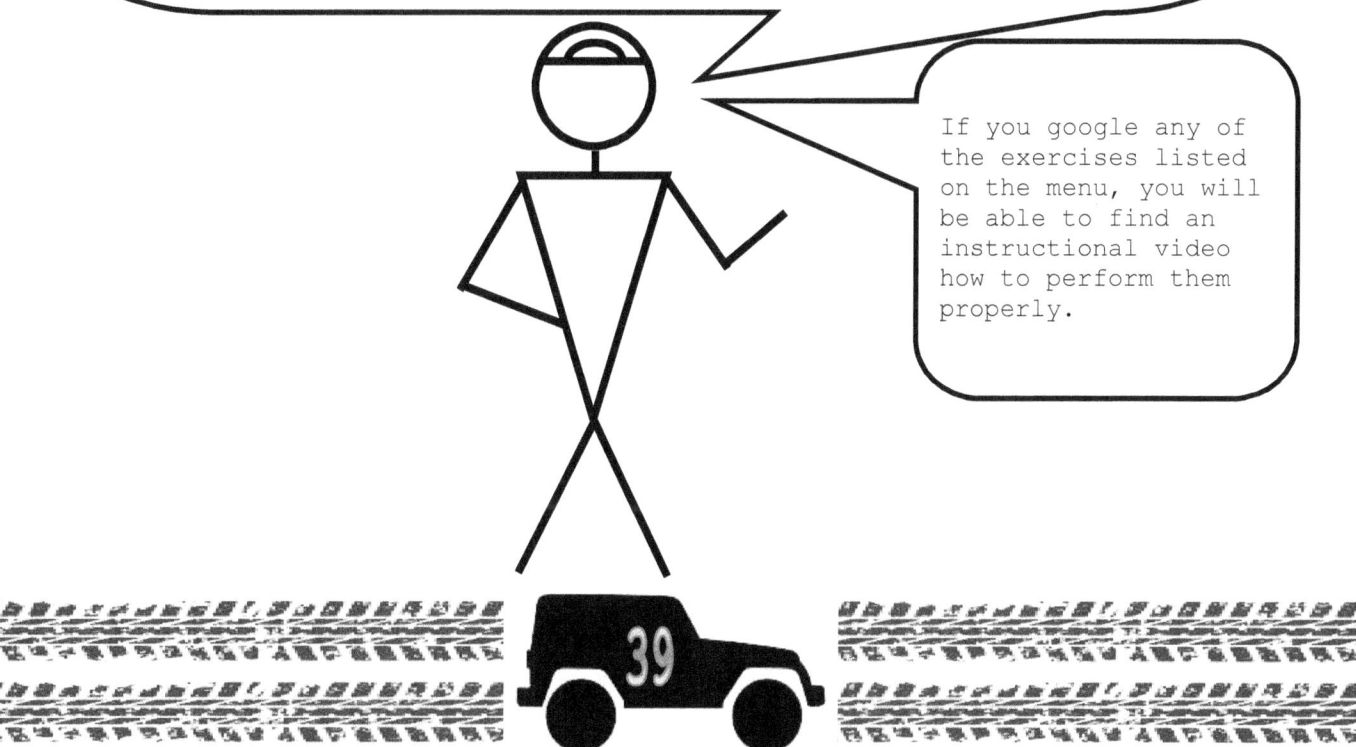

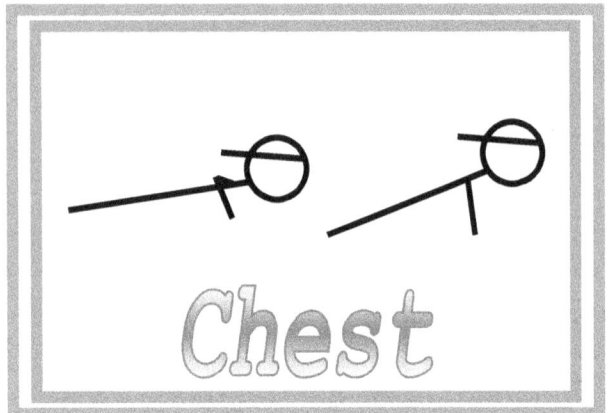

- *Chest Press*
  - Pushups
  - Dumbbells
  - Barbell (bench press)
  - Resistance Band
  - Suspension Trainer
- *Chest Fly*
  - Wide-stance pushups
  - Dumbbells
  - Resistance Band
  - Suspension Trainer

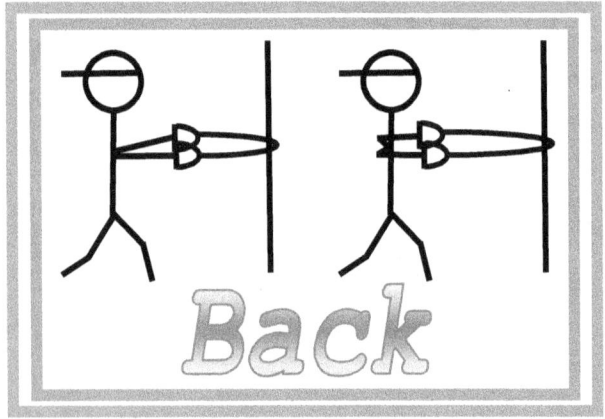

- *Back Row*
  - Dumbbells
  - Barbell
  - Resistance Band
  - Suspension Trainer
- *Back Fly*
  - Dumbbells
  - Resistance Band
  - Suspension Trainer

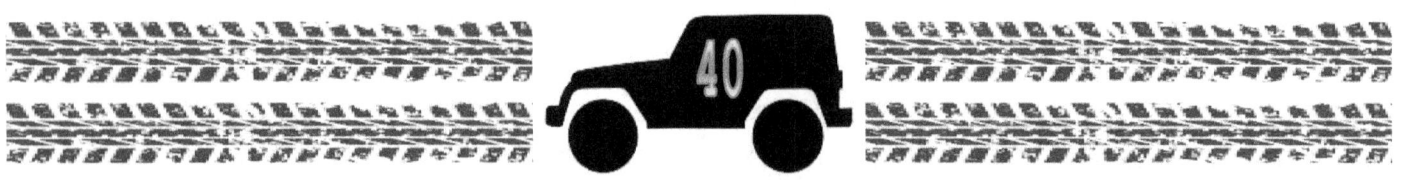

Exercise Menu

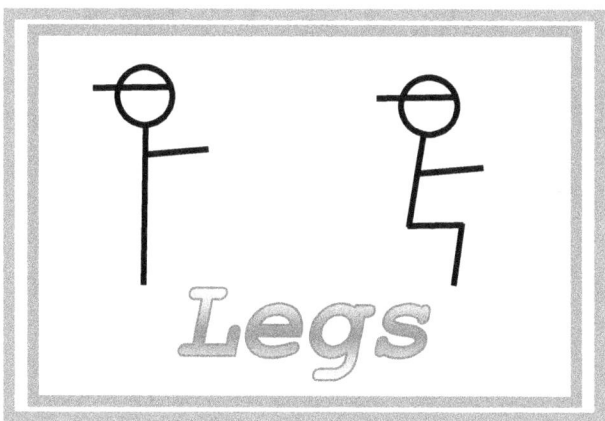

- **Squats**
  - Bodyweight
  - Dumbbells
  - Barbell
  - Medicine Ball
  - Kettlebell
  - Jump Squats
- **Lunges**
  - Walking Lunge
  - Reverse Lunge
  - Side Lunge
  - Jump Lunge

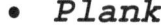

- **Plank**
  - Basic pushup stance
  - Elbows
  - Stability Ball
  - Side-plank
  - Suspension Trainer (feet in straps)
- **Other**
  - Mountain Climbers
  - Reverse Crunch
  - Stability Ball Crunch
  - Scissor Kicks

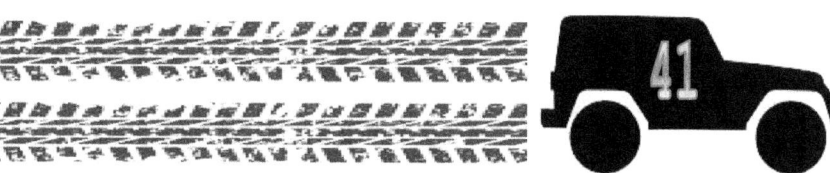
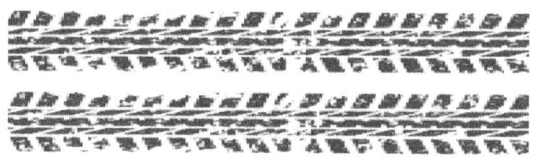

Email: tj@trainingwheelsofwellness.com

Most Requested Body Types

"Light & Lean"

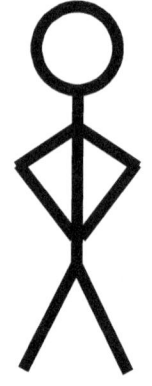

- Built for endurance
- Marathon capable
- Body-weight strength
- Beach-season ready

- 15—25 Reps/exercise
- 3 Sets
- Body-weight training
- Big fan of cardio

"Everyday Rugged"

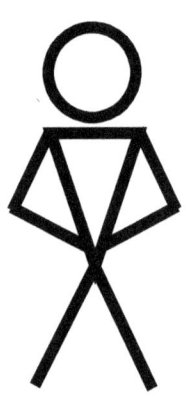

- Built for versatility
- All-sports, 5k, 10k, 1/2 marathon
- Body-weight + Moderate weight strength
- Help-a-friend-move ready

- 12—20 Reps/exercise
- 3 Sets
- Body-weight + Moderate-weight training
- Fan of cardio

"BEAST"

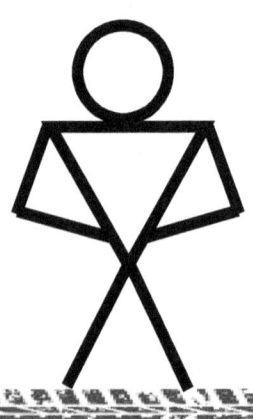

- Built for strength and power
- Running?...not so much
- Heavy-weight strength
- Fire-hydrant-relocation ready

- 6—10 Reps/exercise
- 3 Sets
- Heavy-weight training
- Cardio...meh...not so much

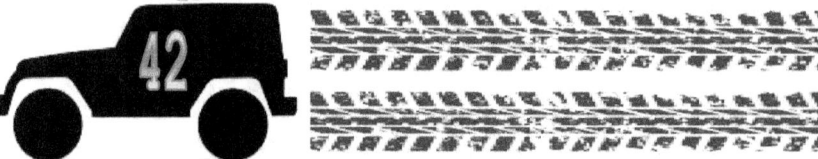

Everyone has their reasons for wanting a certain body-type. More often then not, new clients tend to ask me to make them look like one of the three types listed on the previous page. I challenge them to think beyond the look and focus on the function of the body-type. What activities would you like to be able to do or what capabilities are you seeking? Which body -type makes the most sense for your life now and in the future?

Daily Activities

Weekend Warrior Activities

Hobbies & Sports

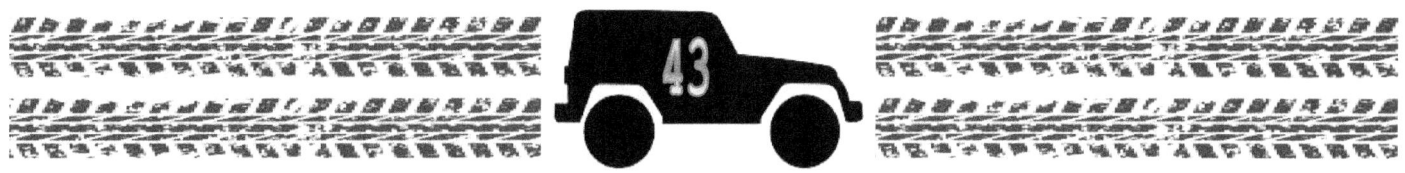

When I first started out as a personal trainer, I would tell my clients to engage in an activity that would slightly elevate their heart rate for 30-60 minutes on the days that they were not doing their circuit training. I called that training "Active Rest" because they were being active but allowing their muscles the opportunity to recover and repair.

Now, we in the fitness industry call that style of training LISS or Low Intensity Steady State training. Basically, you are moving around in a way that causes your heart rate to elevate slightly for an extended period of time of 30-60 minutes.

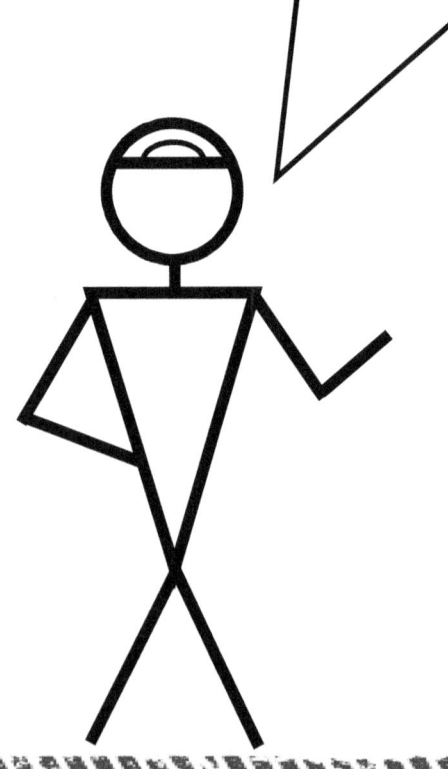

- *Walking*
- *Hiking*
- *Jogging*
- *Biking*
- *Gardening*
- *Housework*
- *Chopping Wood*
- *Canoeing/Kayaking*
- *Swimming*
- *High-intensity board games...?*

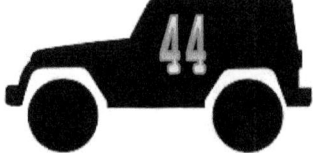
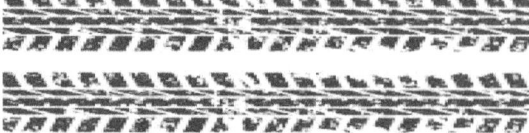

	Monday	Tuesday	Wednesday	Thursday	Friday	Saturday	Sunday
Week 1	Circuit 2 sets	🏃	Circuit 2 sets	🏃	🏃	Circuit 2 sets	Rest
Week 2	🏃	Circuit 2 sets	🏃	Circuit 2 sets	🏃	Circuit 2 sets	Rest
Week 3	Circuit 3 sets	🏃	Circuit 3 sets	🏃	Circuit 3 sets	🏃	Rest
Week 4	Circuit 3 sets	🏃	🏃	Circuit 3 sets	🏃	Circuit 3 sets	Rest

🏃 = **Active Rest AKA LISS training 30-60 minutes!**

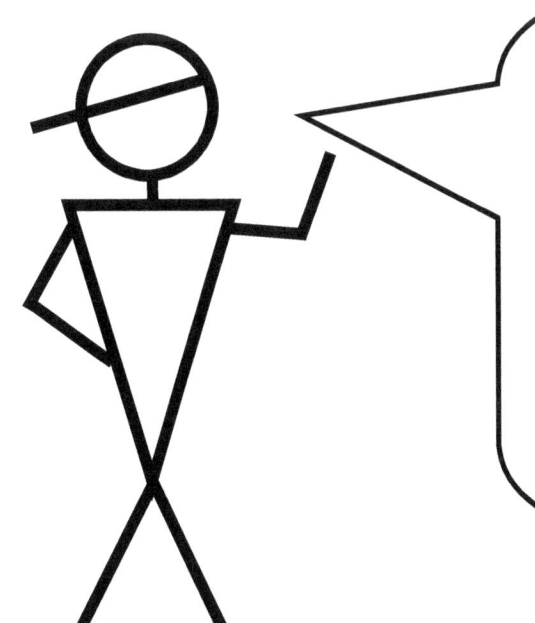

This calendar represents an example of how to approach your month. You can definitely flex the schedule a bit to meet the demands of your week but the goal is to get 3 days of the circuit in and 3 days of other activities that will keep your heartrate elevated for 30-60 minutes. I do recommend spreading out the circuit days throughout the week to allow the muscles to repair themselves before the next circuit day.

Also, be sure to take a rest day during each week to give your body a chance to rest. Resting tips will be covered in the next section.

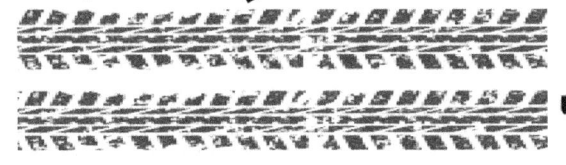
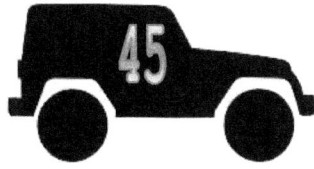
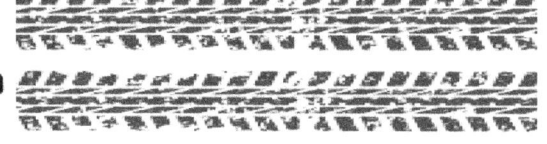

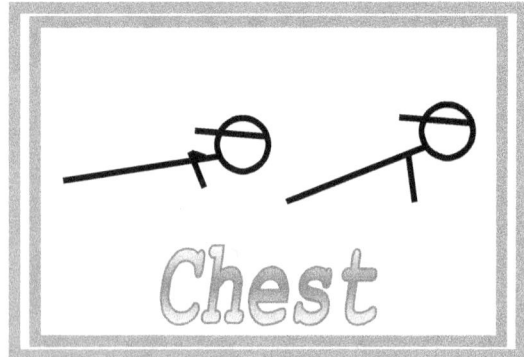

Exercise 1:

Exercise 2:

Exercise 3:

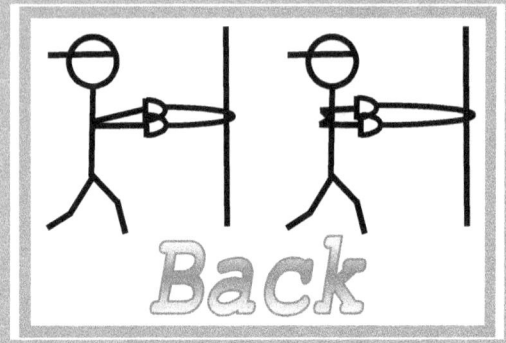

Exercise 1:

Exercise 2:

Exercise 3:

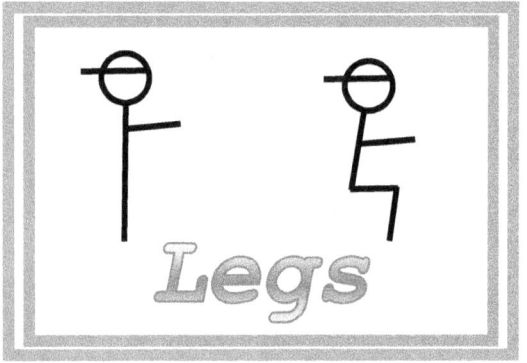

Exercise 1:

Exercise 2:

Exercise 3:

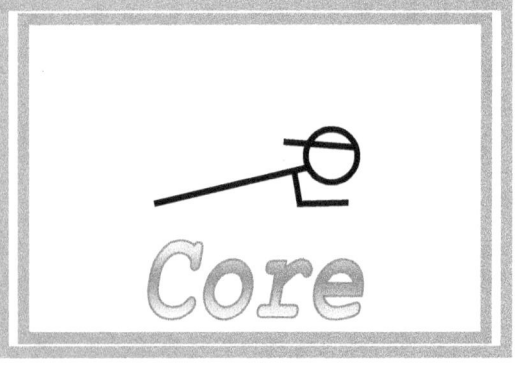

Exercise 1:

Exercise 2:

Exercise 3:

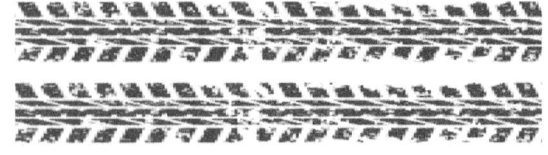

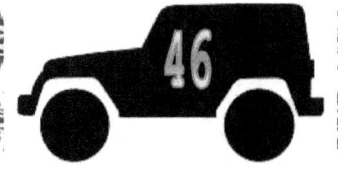

Month 1

	Monday	Tuesday	Wednesday	Thursday	Friday	Saturday	Sunday
Week 1							
Week 2							
Week 3							
Week 4							

Month 2

	Monday	Tuesday	Wednesday	Thursday	Friday	Saturday	Sunday
Week 1							
Week 2							
Week 3							
Week 4							

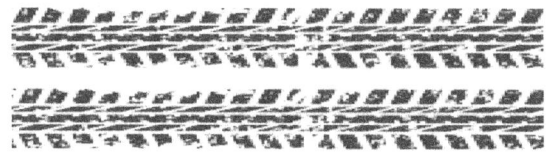 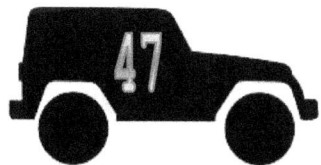 

At this time, I would like to introduce you to one of the greatest pieces of equipment of all time. Say hello to the rowing machine!

I recommend this larger piece of equipment above all others because of its versatility and return on "sweat investment".

Need an excellent warm-up? Hop on the rower.

Need a quick workout that will blast more muscle groups than any other piece of cardio equipment? Hop on the rower.

Interval training? Rower.

Cool down? Rower.

LISS training? Rower.

Rehabilitating? Rower.

Get it?

My all-time favorite rower is the Concept 2 Model D. It is a solid piece of equipment that does not require a lot of maintenance and will stand the test of time in your home gym.

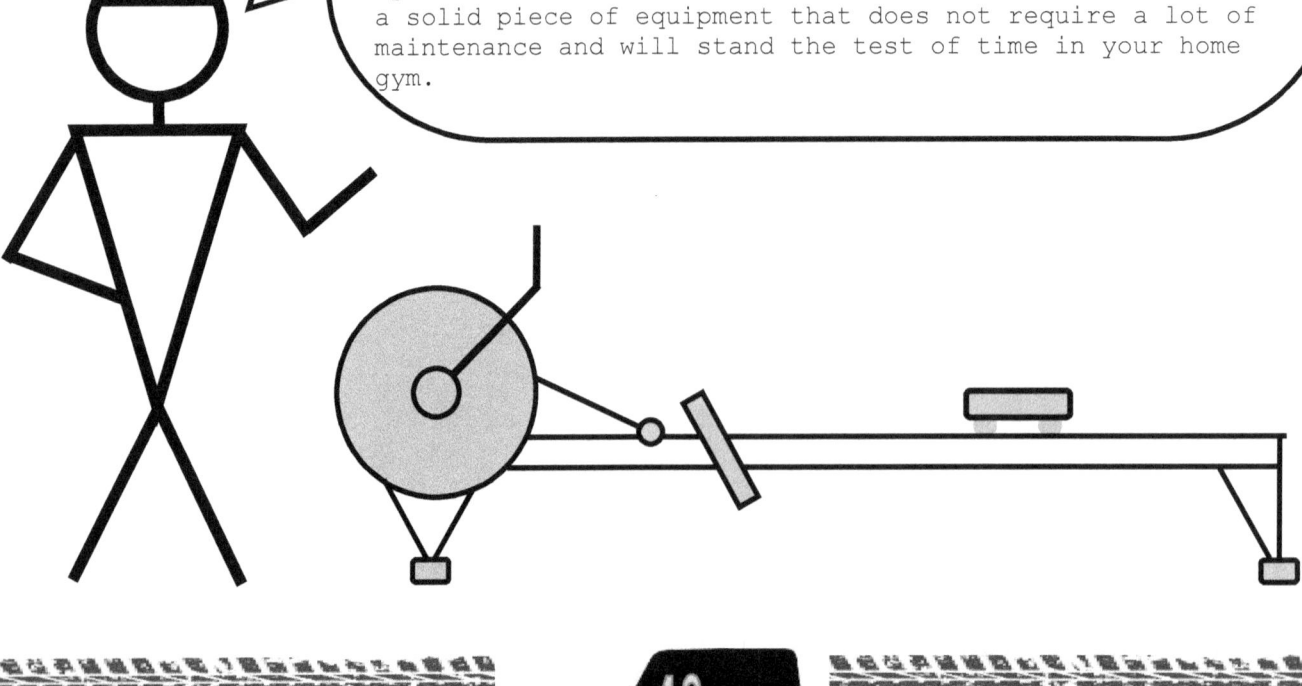

Resistance Bands

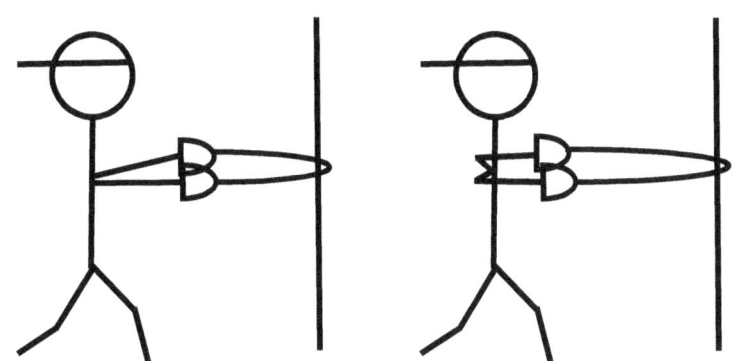

Suspension Trainer

I am a huge fan of versatility and efficiency which is why I recommend these pieces of equipment. Whenever I have to travel, these are the pieces of equipment that make the trip with me. They are inexpensive but can be used for so many different exercises, can be set up easily, and take up very little space.

For the resistance bands, I recommend SPRI braided bands because of their durability.

As for choosing a suspension trainer, I recommend the WOSS trainer. It's made in the USA and very affordable.

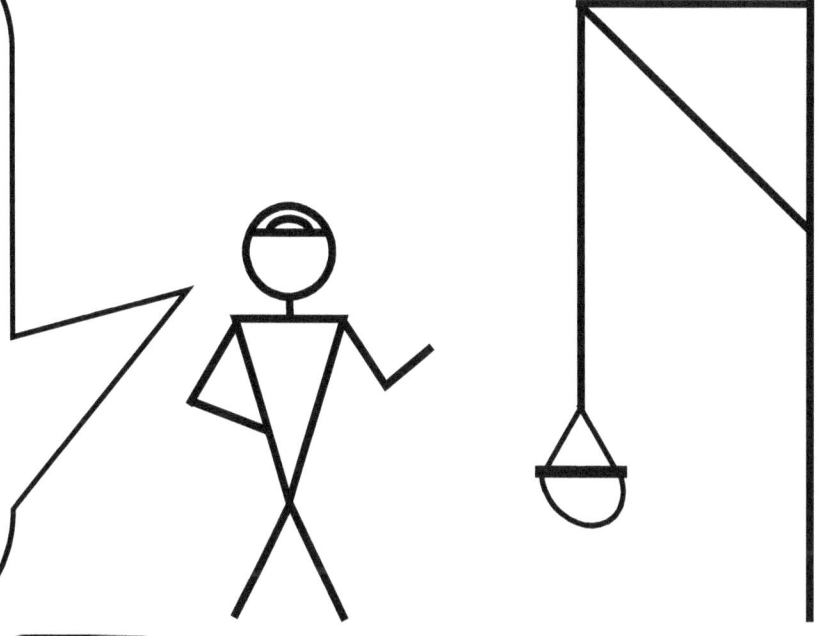

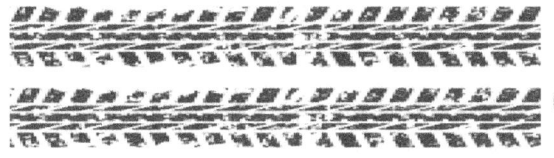
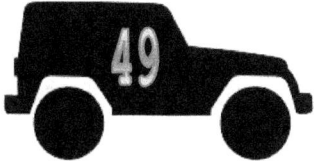
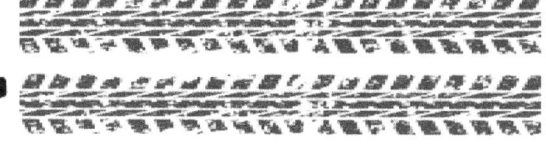

For further reflection and information:

- http://blog.nasm.org

- http://healthandsociety.com/journal

- https://www.myfitnesspal.com

- http://www.mapmyrun.com

- https://www.outsideonline.com/fitness

- http://www.naturalmuscle.net

- http://www.chrismcdougall.com

- https://www.nsca.com/uploadedFiles/NSCA/Resources/PDF/Education/ Tools_and_Resources/FoundationsofFitnessProgramming_201508.pdf

- http://www.concept2.com/indoor-rowers/model-d

- http://www.woss.com/woss-trainers

- http://www.spri.com/braided-tubing

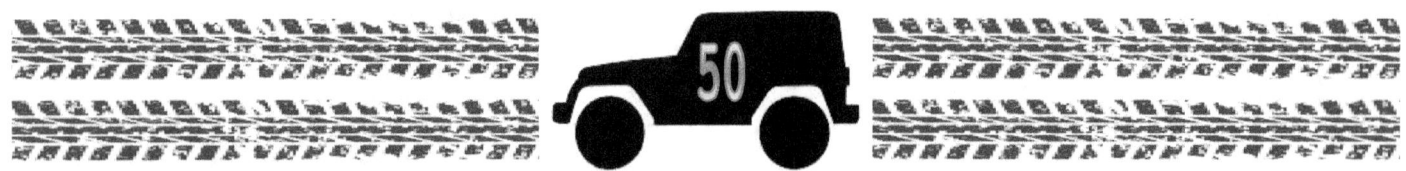

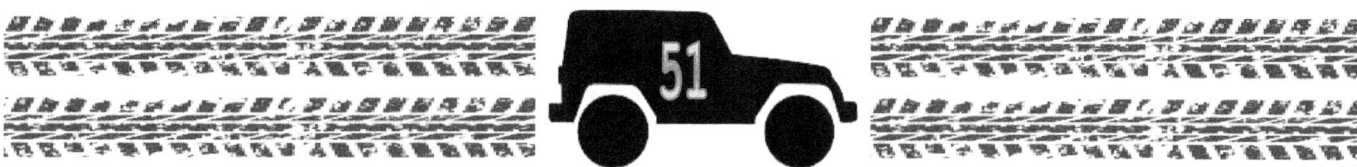

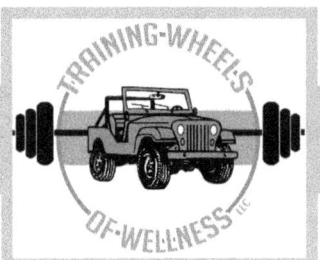

Part 4: Rest

When you train, you cause small tears in your muscle fibers and this type of stress damage is actually a good thing. Your body will start repairing the muscle fibers immediately after you end your training session. If you continually stress these muscle fibers in a particular way, the body will repair the muscle fibers to meet these new demands because the body is amazing.

In addition to proper nutrition, resting the body allows for quality recovery.

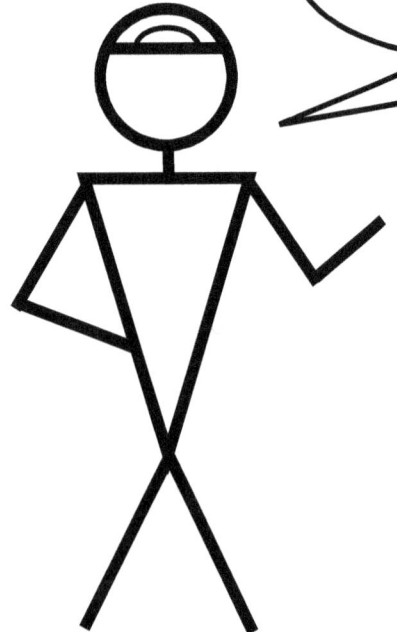

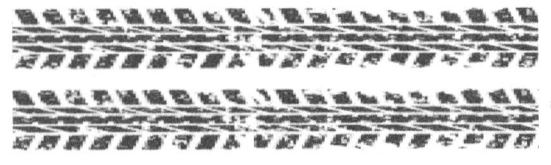
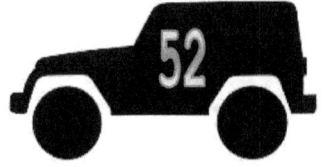
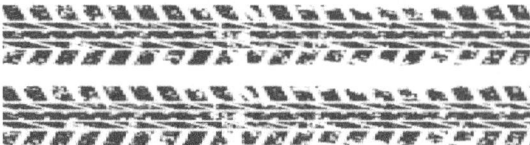

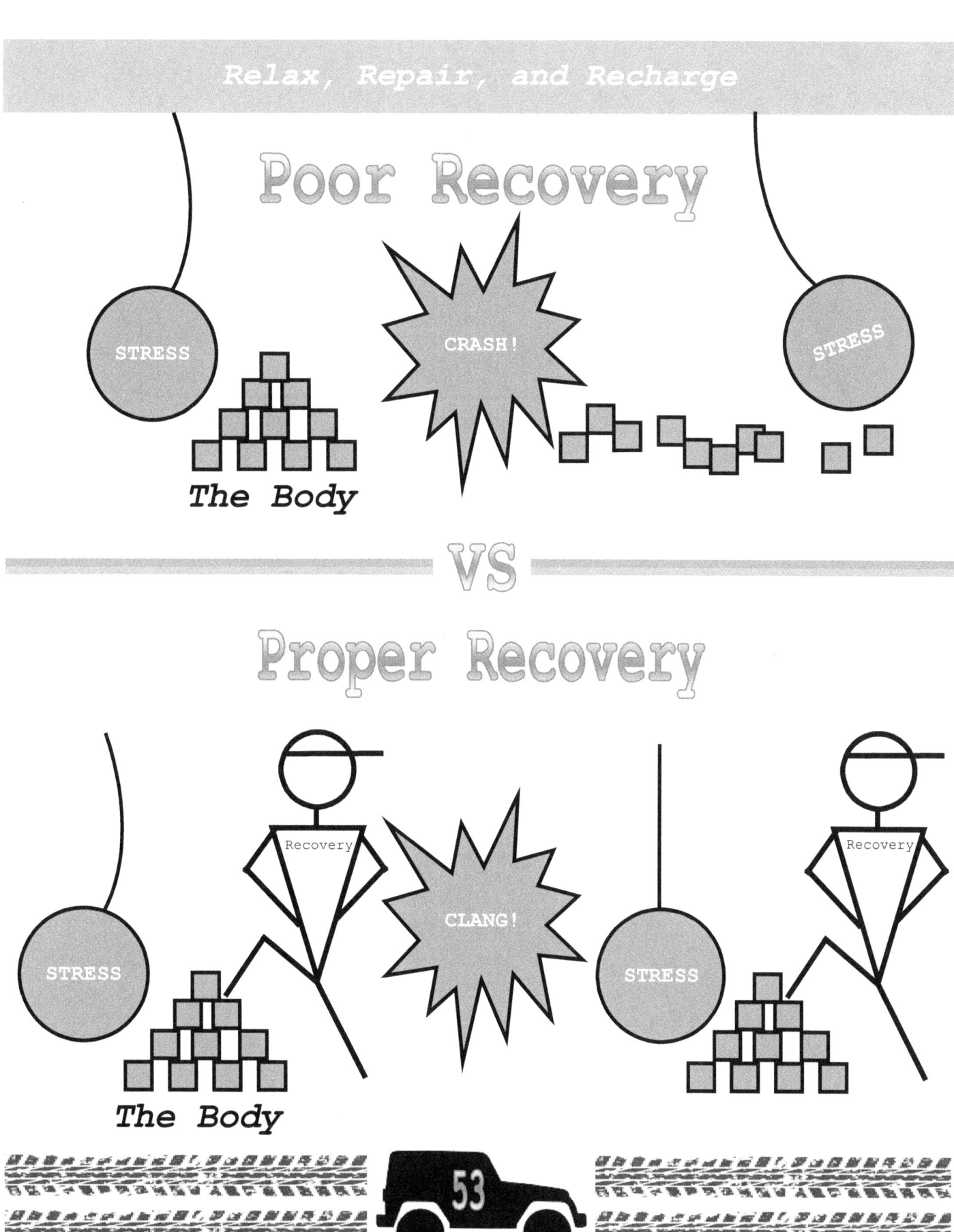

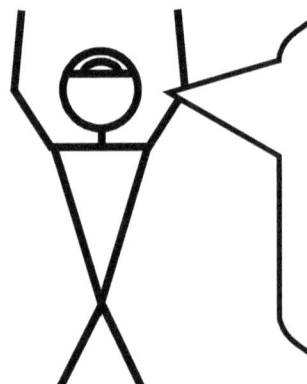

Raise your hand if you like naps! I have two hands up because of how much I enjoy napping.
I may not pass out for the whole nap. Sometimes I just lay there with my feet up and my eyes closed to allow my mind wander for the 25 minutes. When my timer goes off, I stand up, stretch, and feel rejuvenated to take on the rest of my day.

Naps are fantastic and I recommend the following steps for a successful nap:

Step 1: Set a Timer
00:25:00

Step 2: Get Comfortable

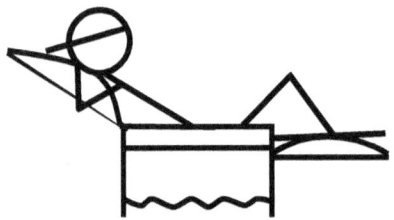

Step 3: Doze away!

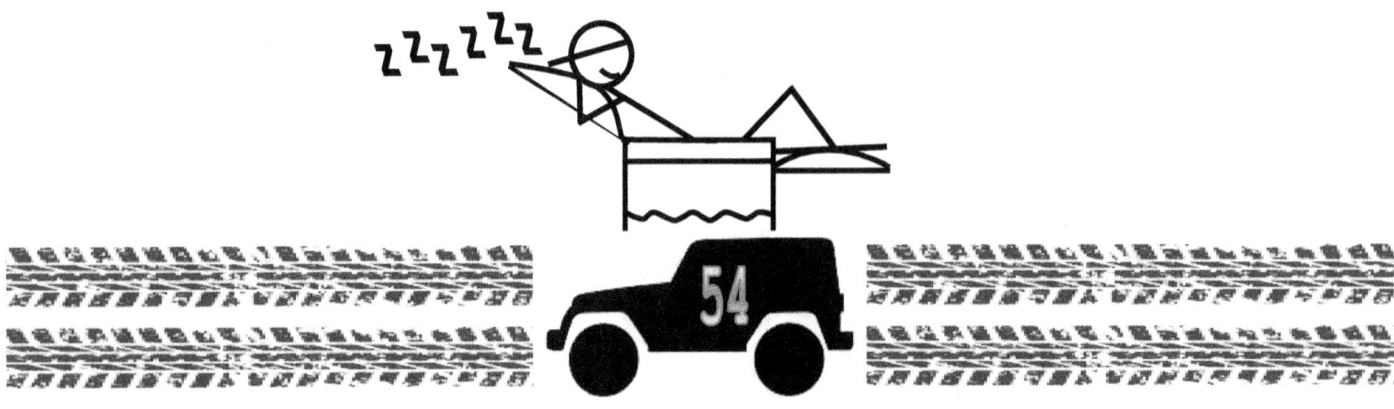

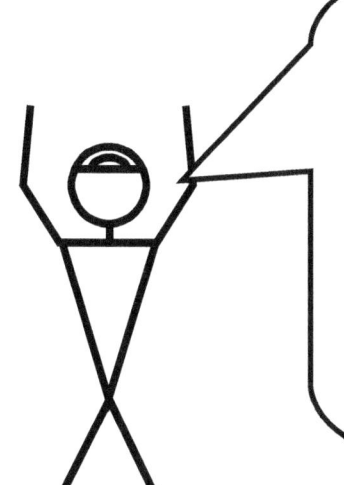

YUP! I still have my hands up because I love sleep THAT much! Everyone's sleeping pattern is unique so I encourage each person I work with to experiment with different sleep times to see which amount of sleep works best for them.

For some, 6 hours works wonders and they wake up fully refreshed. For others, it's 8 hours. Basically, your sleep amount should provide you with energy to take on the day. If you are waking up feeling sleep deprived, you clearly need more sleep!

Below are some helpful hints to give you a chance at a better night's sleep.

- If you are able to, set the temperature to 66-68 degrees.

- Stop looking at anything with a screen 1-2 hours before your planned bedtime.

- Charge your phone on the other side of the room.

- Read a book...like an actual book.

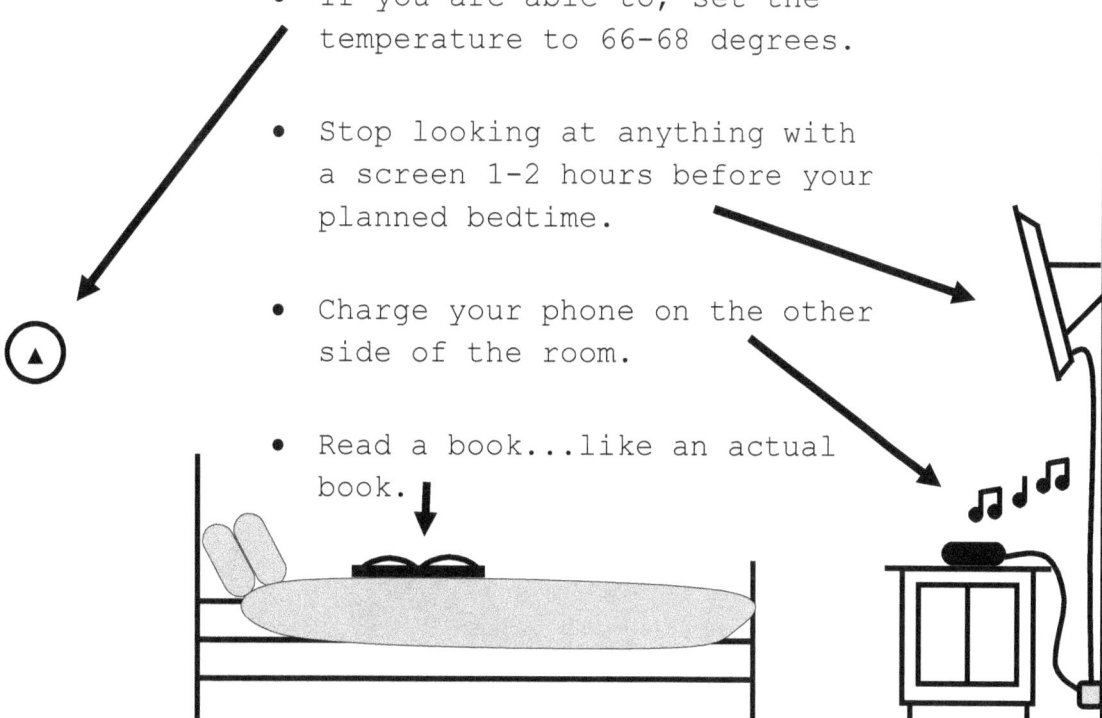

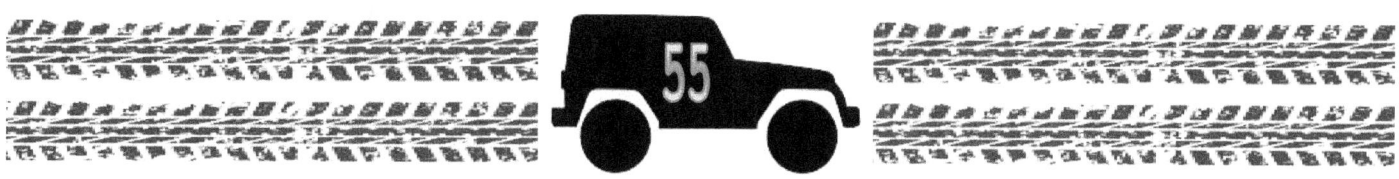

For further reflection and information:

- *https://sleepfoundation.org/*

- *http://greatist.com/*

- *http://www.journalsleep.org/Default.aspx*

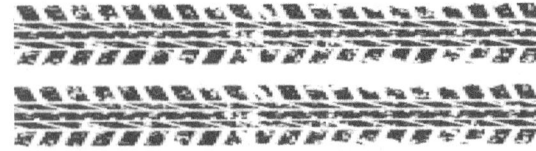
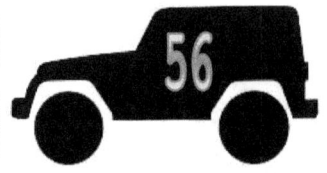

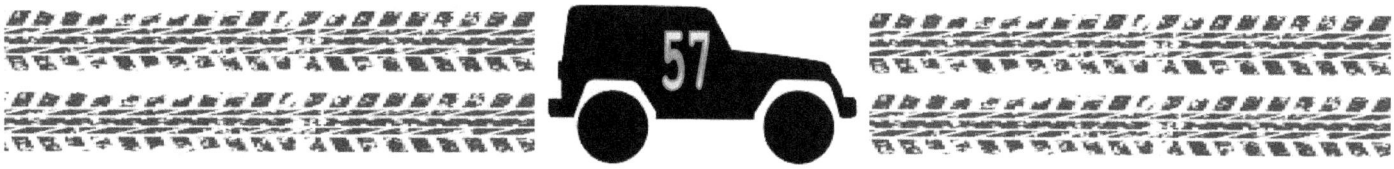

Life

- From Huntington, New York
- Grew up running around in the neighborhood and playing soccer
- Lost 70 pounds while going to SUNY Albany
- Lived and worked in California for an Outdoor Education facility from 2007-2011
- Lived, learned, and worked in Wisconsin from 2011-2014
- Returned to New York in 2014 to help others with their health and wellness by starting Training Wheels of Wellness LLC
- Enjoys laughing with friends and family, reading, circuit training, biking, hiking, exploring, camping, educating, tinkering, all things Jeep, and volunteering

> *"Life is 10% what happens to you and 90% how you react to it." - Charles Swindoll*

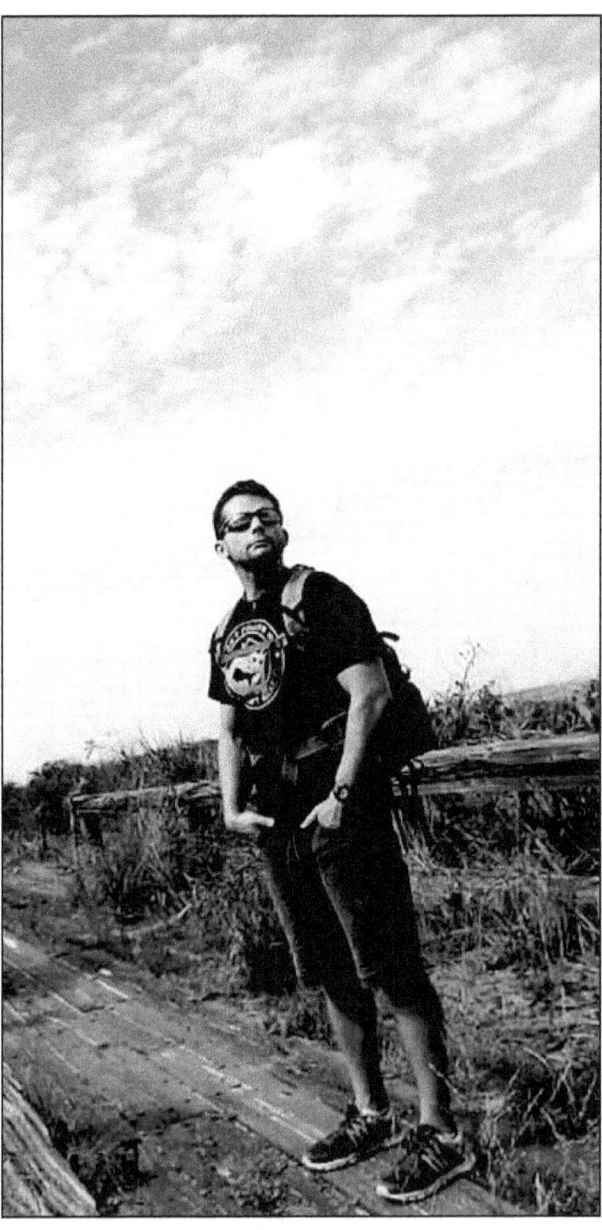

Education

- BA Sociology: SUNY Albany
- MS Recreation Administration: George Williams College of Aurora University

Certifications

- Certified Personal Trainer (CPT):
- Fitness Nutrition Specialist (FNS)
- MMA Conditioning Specialist (MMACS)
- Youth Exercise Specialist (YES)

National Academy of Sports Medicine (NASM)

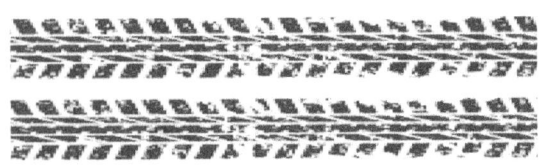
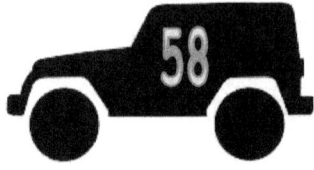
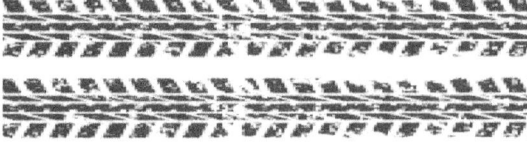

Once upon a time...

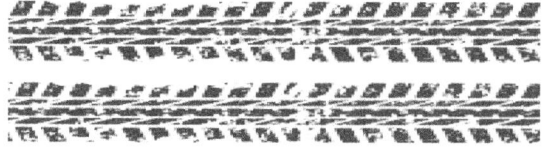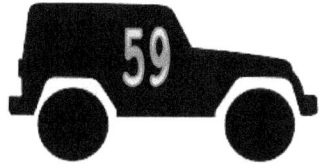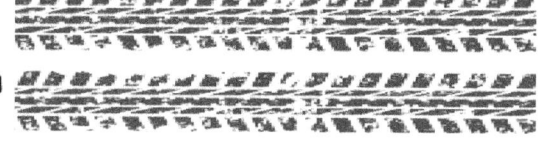